PERIPHERAL NERVE BLOCKS

and PERI-OPERATIVE PAIN RELIEF

ELSEVIER DVD-ROM LICENCE AGREEMENT

PLEASE READ THE FOLLOWING AGREEMENT CAREFULLY BEFORE USING THIS PRODUCT. THIS PRODUCT IS LICENSED UNDER THE TERMS CONTAINED IN THIS LICENCE AGREE-MENT ('Agreement'). BY USING THIS PRODUCT, YOU, AN INDIVIDUAL OR ENTITY INCLUDING EMPLOYEES, AGENTS AND REPRESENTATIVES ('You' or 'Your'), ACKNOWLEDGE THAT YOU HAVE READ THIS AGREEMENT, THAT YOU UNDERSTAND IT, AND THAT YOU AGREE TO BE BOUND BY THE TERMS AND CONDITIONS OF THIS AGREEMENT. ELSEVIER LIMITED ('Elsevier') EXPRESSLY DOES NOT AGREE TO LICENSE THIS PRODUCT TO YOU UNLESS YOU ASSENT TO THIS AGREEMENT. IF YOU DO NOT AGREE WITH ANY OF THE FOLLOWING TERMS, YOU MAY, WITHIN THIRTY (30) DAYS AFTER YOUR RECEIPT OF THIS PRODUCT RETURN THE UNUSED PRODUCT AND ALL ACCOMPANYING DOCUMENTATION TO ELSEVIER FOR A FULL REFUND.

DEFINITIONS As used in this Agreement, these terms shall have the following meanings:

'Proprietary Material' means the valuable and proprietary information content of this Product including without limitation all indexes and graphic materials and software used to access, index, search and retrieve the information content from this Product developed or licensed by Elsevier and/or its affiliates, suppliers and licensors.

'Product' means the copy of the Proprietary Material and any other material delivered on DVD-ROM and any other human-readable or machine-readable materials enclosed with this Agreement, including without limitation documentation relating to the same.

OWNERSHIP This Product has been supplied by and is proprietary to Elsevier and/or its affiliates, suppliers and licensors. The copyright in the Product belongs to Elsevier and/or its affiliates, suppliers and licensors and is protected by the copyright, trademark, trade secret and other intellectual property laws of the United Kingdom and international treaty provisions, including without limitation the Universal Copyright Convention and the Berne Copyright Convention. You have no ownership rights in this Product. Except as expressly set forth herein, no part of this Product, including without limitation the Proprietary Material, may be modified, copied or distributed in hardcopy or machine-readable form without prior written consent from Elsevier. All rights not expressly granted to You herein are expressly reserved. Any other use of this Product by any person or entity is strictly prohibited and a violation of this Agreement.

SCOPE OF RIGHTS LICENSED (PERMITTED USES) Elsevier is granting to You a limited, non-exclusive, non-transferable licence to use this Product in accordance with the terms of this Agreement. You may use or provide access to this Product on a single computer or terminal physically located at Your premises and in a secure network or move this Product to and use it on another single computer or terminal at the same location for personal use only, but under no circumstances may You use or provide access to any part or parts of this Product on more than one computer or terminal simultaneously.

You shall not (a) copy, download, or otherwise reproduce the Product or any part(s) thereof in any medium, including, without limitation, online transmissions, local area networks, wide area networks, intranets, extranets and the Internet, or in any way, in whole or in part, except for printing out or downloading nonsubstantial portions of the text and images in the Product for Your own personal use; (b) alter, modify, or adapt the Product or any part(s) thereof, including but not limited to decompiling, disassembling, reverse engineering, or creating derivative works, without the prior written approval of Elsevier; (c) sell, license or otherwise distribute to third parties the Product or any part(s) thereof; or (d) alter, remove, obscure or obstruct the display of any copyright, trademark or other proprietary notice on or in the Product or on any printout or download of portions of the Proprietary Materials.

Restrictions on Transfer This Licence is personal to You, and neither Your rights hereunder nor the tangible embodiments of this Product, including without limitation the Proprietary Material, may be sold, assigned, transferred or sublicensed to any other person, including without limitation by operation of law, without the prior written consent of Elsevier. Any purported sale, assignment, transfer or sublicense without the prior written consent of Elsevier will be void and will automatically terminate the Licence granted hereunder.

TERM This Agreement will remain in effect until terminated pursuant to the terms of this Agreement. You may terminate this Agreement at any time by removing from Your system and destroying the Product and any copies of the Proprietary Material. Unauthorized copying of the Product, including without limitation, the Proprietary Material and documentation, or otherwise failing to comply with the terms and conditions of this Agreement shall result in automatic termination of this licence and will make available to Elsevier legal remedies. Upon termination of this Agreement, the licence granted herein will terminate and You must immediately destroy the Product and all copies of the Product and of the Proprietary Material, together with any and all accompanying documentation. All provisions relating to proprietary rights shall survive termination of this Agreement.

LIMITED WARRANTY AND LIMITATION OF LIABILITY Elsevier warrants that the software embodied in this Product will perform in substantial compliance with the documentation supplied in this Product, unless the performance problems are the result of hardware failure or improper use. If You report a significant defect in performance in writing to Elsevier within ninety (90) calendar days of your having purchased the Product, and Elsevier is not able to correct same within sixty (60) days after its receipt of Your notification, You may return this Product, including all copies and documentation, to Elsevier and Elsevier will refund Your money. In order to apply for a refund on your purchased Product, please contact the return address on the invoice to obtain the refund request form ('Refund Request Form'), and either fax or mail your signed request and your proof of purchase to the address indicated on the Refund Request Form. Incomplete forms will not be processed. Defined terms in the Refund Request Form shall have the same meaning as in this Agreement.

YOU UNDERSTAND THAT, EXCEPT FOR THE LIMITED WARRANTY RECITED ABOVE, ELSEVIER, ITS AFFILIATES, LICENSORS, THIRD PARTY SUPPLIERS AND AGENTS (TOGETHER 'THE SUPPLIERS') MAKE NO REPRESENTATIONS OR WARRANTIES, WITH RESPECT TO THE PRODUCT, INCLUDING, WITHOUT LIMITATION THE PROPRIETARY MATERIAL. ALL OTHER REPRESENTATIONS, WARRANTIES, CONDITIONS OR OTHER TERMS, WHETHER EXPRESS OR IMPLIED BY STATUTE OR COMMON LAW, ARE HEREBY EXCLUDED TO THE FULLEST EXTENT PERMITTED BY LAW.

IN PARTICULAR BUT WITHOUT LIMITATION TO THE FOREGOING NONE OF THE SUPPLIERS MAKE ANY REPRESENTATIONS OR WARRANTIES (WHETHER EXPRESS OR IMPLIED) REGARDING THE PERFORMANCE OF YOUR PAD, NETWORK OR COMPUTER SYSTEM WHEN USED IN CONJUNCTION WITH THE PRODUCT, NOR THAT THE PRODUCT WILL MEET YOUR REQUIREMENTS OR THAT ITS OPERATION WILL BE UNINTERRUPTED OR ERROR-FREE.

EXCEPT IN RESPECT OF DEATH OR PERSONAL INJURY CAUSED BY THE SUPPLIERS' NEGLIGENCE AND TO THE FULLEST EXTENT PERMITTED BY LAW, IN NO EVENT (AND REGARDLESS OF WHETHER SUCH DAMAGES ARE FORESEEABLE AND OF WHETHER SUCH LIABILITY IS BASED IN TORT, CONTRACT OR OTHERWISE) WILL ANY OF THE SUPPLIERS BE LIABLE TO YOU FOR ANY DAMAGES (INCLUDING, WITHOUT LIMITATION, ANY LOST PROFITS, LOST SAVINGS OR OTHER SPECIAL, INDIRECT, INCIDENTAL OR CONSEQUENTIAL DAMAGES ARISING OUT OF OR RESULTING FROM: (I) YOUR USE OF, OR INABILITY TO USE, THE PRODUCT; (II) DATA LOSS OR CORRUPTION; AND/OR (III) ERRORS OR OMISSIONS IN THE PROPRIETARY MATERIAL.

IF THE FOREGOING LIMITATION IS HELD TO BE UNENFORCEABLE, OUR MAXIMUM LIABILITY TO YOU IN RESPECT THEREOF SHALL NOT EXCEED THE AMOUNT OF THE LICENCE FEE PAID BY YOU FOR THE PRODUCT. THE REMEDIES AVAILABLE TO YOU AGAINST ELSEVIER AND THE LICENSORS OF MATERIALS INCLUDED IN THE PRODUCT ARE EXCLUSIVE.

If the information provided in the Product contains medical or health sciences information, it is intended for professional use within the medical field. Information about medical treatment or drug dosages is intended strictly for professional use, and because of rapid advances in the medical sciences, independent verification of diagnosis and drug dosages should be made.

The provisions of this Agreement shall be severable, and in the event that any provision of this Agreement is found to be legally unenforceable, such unenforceability shall not prevent the enforcement or any other provision of this Agreement.

GOVERNING LAW This Agreement shall be governed by the laws of England and Wales. In any dispute arising out of this Agreement, you and Elsevier each consent to the exclusive personal jurisdiction and venue in the courts of England and Wales.

PERIPHERAL NERVE BLOCKS

and PERI-OPERATIVE PAIN RELIEF

Jack Barrett FFARCS(I) Dip. Pain Medicine
Consultant Anaesthetist
Department of Anaesthesia and Intensive Care Medicine
University College Cork
Cork University Hospital
Cork, Ireland

Dominic Harmon FFARCS(I) FRCA
Specialist Registrar in Anaesthesia
Department of Anaesthesia and Intensive Care Medicine
University College Cork
Cork University Hospital
Cork, Ireland

Frank Loughnane FCA(RCSI)
Specialist Registrar in Anaesthesia
Department of Anaesthesia and Intensive Care Medicine
University College Cork
Cork University Hospital
Cork, Ireland

Brendan Finucane FRCA FRCP(C)
Professor and Residency Program Director
Department of Anesthesiology and Pain Medicine
University of Alberta
Edmonton, Alberta, Canada

George Shorten FFARCS(I) FRCA MD PhD
Professor of Anaesthesia and Intensive Care Medicine
Department of Anaesthesia and Intensive Care Medicine
University College Cork
Cork University Hospital
Cork, Ireland

SAUNDERS

Edinburgh • London • New York • Oxford • Philadelphia • St Louis • Sydney • Toronto 2004

SAUNDERS
An imprint of Elsevier Limited

First published 2004
  Reprinted 2005

ISBN 0 7020 2717 0

British Library Cataloguing in Publication Data
A catalogue record for this book is available from the British Library

Library of Congress Cataloguing in Publication Data
A catalogue record for this book is available from the Library of Congress

Notice
Medical knowledge is constantly changing. Standard safety precautions
must be followed, but as new research and clinical experience broaden
our knowledge, changes in treatment and drug therapy may become
necessary r appropriate. Readers are advised to check the most current
product information provided by the manufactacturer of each drug to be
administered to verify the recommended dose, the method and duration
of administration, and contraindications. It is the responsibility of the
practitioner, relying on experience and knowledge of the patient, to
determine dosages and the best treatment for each individual patient.
Neither the Publisher nor the editors assume any liability for any injury
and/or damage to persons or property arising from this publication.

The Publisher

Commissioning Editor: Paul Fam
Project Development Manager: Shuet-Kei Cheung
Project Manager: Rory MacDonald
Illustration Manager: Mick Ruddy
Design Direction: Andy Chapman
Illustrator: Mark Willey

Printed in China

Last digit is print number 9 8 7 6 5 4 3 2

The
publisher's
policy is to use
**paper manufactured
from sustainable forests**

Contents

Foreword

Regional anesthesia has come to stay. Its development and progress have been slow, principally because the anesthetist must have an accurate knowledge of anatomy and a high degree of technical skill in order that the anesthesia may be safe and satisfactory, and that the operation not delayed.' These words by surgeon William J. Mayo opened the foreword to Gaston Labat's *Regional Anesthesia, Its Technic and Application*[1]. Published in 1922, Labat's text focused on the perioperative management of patients undergoing intra-abdominal, head and neck, and extremity procedures using infiltration, peripheral, plexus, and splanchnic blockade (using recently introduced procaine); neuraxial techniques were not widely applied at the time.

The art and science of regional anesthesia have progressed significantly over the last century, resulting in improved safety and increased success rates. The frequency of serious complications related to neural blockade continues to decrease and is similar, if not superior, to that of general anesthesia. Improved methods of neural localization and imaging such as fluoroscopy, high-resolution ultrasound and stimulating catheters have facilitated accurate needle/catheter placement.

Most importantly, prospective randomized clinical investigations have demonstrated improved outcomes for patients undergoing major surgical procedures when regional anesthesia and analgesia is utilized. Thus, issues regarding safety, success rate, and efficacy have been addressed.

However, it is noteworthy that several of the early concerns have changed little. For example, an understanding of anatomic relationships, neural innervation, and physiology remain paramount in the application of regional anesthetic and analgesic techniques. Many clinicians do not have ready access to an anatomy laboratory and classic anatomical atlases were constructed by anatomists, not regional anesthesiologists, resulting in illustrations that depict neural anatomy with the 'wrong' limb orientation and/or cross-sectional view. Finally, the majority of resident training programs do not provide formal training in peripheral blockade. Experienced clinicians and trainees must both have access to anatomic sections and simulators, allowing the proceduralist to explore the anatomical relationships between nerves and related structures prior to patient contact.

From this perspective, I have found the content, organization, and multimedia components of *Peripheral Nerve Blocks and Perioperative Pain Relief* both thorough and comprehensive. The authors present the superficial and deep anatomical relationships using text, line drawings, still photographs, MR images, and video clips. The block techniques themselves are depicted in still photographs and video demonstrations, often with associated MR images of local anesthetic distribution. Thus, the text and DVD-ROM complement each other and provide the reader with a knowledge base that builds on itself to describe safe, efficacious and efficient peripheral blockade.

Labat[1] concluded in his 1922 text, 'Regional anesthesia is an art.' Nearly a century later, *Peripheral Nerve Blocks and Perioperative Pain Relief* characterizes the current state of the art (and science) of regional anesthesia. I applaud the authors for their accomplishment.

References
Labat G. Regional Anesthesia: Its Technic and Clinical Application. Philadelphia, W. B. Saunders, 1922.

Terese T Horlocker MD

Professor of Anesthesiology
Mayo Clinic College of Medicine
Rochester, MN, USA

President
American Society of Regional Anesthesia and Pain Medicine

Preface

For the past four years, several of the editors of this textbook who are anesthesiologists at Cork University Hospital in Ireland, have organised cadaver-based workshops on peripheral nerve blockade (PNB). The intent was to provide a detailed foundation upon which clinicians might develop their expertise in PNB. We were impressed by the number and enthusiasm of those who attended. It was clear that many anesthesiologists (and other specialists) were keen to learn or refresh their knowledge of the subject.

One principle became abundantly clear as we reviewed the feedback (from both instructors and students) on the course. A thorough understanding of both surface and internal anatomy is essential for the safe and effective performance of peripheral nerve blockade. Although the use of cadaver specimens and human volunteers to illustrate anatomy were useful, we began to use magnetic resonance images (obtained using an 'open' or interventional MR scanner) to study the relevant 'live' anatomy and the spread of injectate. We found these images to have great educational value.

A second observation which consistently appeared in our course reviews was that certain topics were poorly understood or needed to be relearned for application to PNB. These included the basic pharmacology of local anaesthetics, indications/contraindications and complications of PNB and the principles underlying the use of the peripheral nerve stimulator. Although information of these topics was available from various different sources, it seemed reasonable to present the theoretical and practical aspects of PNB as 'a package' comprising three elements: textbook, DVD-ROM and website.

We hope that what has resulted is a 'stand-alone', effective educational tool (comprising textbook, DVD-ROM and web site) which will enable anesthesiologists to learn and practice PNB safely and effectively.

Jack Barrett
Dominic Harmon
Frank Loughane
Brendan Finucane
George Shorten
2004

Acknowledgements

Production costs were sponsored by Abbott Laboratories, Ireland Ltd and B Braun Medical Ltd. The patient and consistent support of Ms Fiona Burke, Manager, Hospital Products Division (Abbott Laboratories) and Dr Martin Sippel, Vice-President, Strategic Marketing (B Braun Melsungen AG) was essential to the successful completion of the project. Thanks are also due to I-Flow Corporation.

The authors also wish to acknowledge the following for their advice, support and hard work in assembling the material contained in this book.

Professor John Fraher, Professor of Anatomy, University College Cork, Ireland for facilitating the preparation of the cadaver dissections (Mr Paul Dansie) and allowing use of his department for the video production of cadaver anatomy.

Mr Aidan Maguire, Television Director for Video Production, and his team comprising Dr Tony Healy and Mr Gerry Ryan.

Mr Peter Murphy, Manager, Open MRI Centre, Cork for producing, labelling and editing the MR images. The proprietors of the Open MRI Centre and the Victoria/South Infirmary Hospital, Cork, Ireland for use of their facility.

Dr Michelle Reardon, Lecturer in Anatomy, University College Cork, Ireland for her advice and assistance with both cadaver and MR anatomy.

Mr Tomás Tyner for his excellent, still photography and Mr Tony Perrott Director of the Department of Audio-Visual Services at University College Cork, Ireland.

All the Volunteers who so willingly made themselves available to have the blocks performed on them for both video and MRI.

Dr John McAdoo, Consultant Anaesthetist, Cork University Hospital, Cork, Ireland for his meticulous contributions (both demonstration and written) on ophthalmic blocks.

Part 1

Principles

CHAPTER 1

Introduction

Within anesthetic practice, the role of regional anesthesia—including peripheral nerve block—has expanded greatly over the past two decades. In 1998, a national survey demonstrated that 87.8% of US anesthesiologists make use of regional techniques.[1] This widespread use arises in part from the widely held belief (to some extent evidence-based) that, at least in some settings, anesthetic techniques that avoid general anesthesia offer real advantages in terms of patient outcome.[2] For instance, Chelly and colleagues have demonstrated clearly that continuous femoral infusion of ropivacaine 0.2% in patients undergoing total knee replacement provides better postoperative analgesia than epidural or patient-controlled analgesia. Critically, this technique accelerated early functional recovery and was associated with decreased duration of hospital stay, postoperative blood loss, and incidence of serious postoperative complications.[3]

A second reason that accounts for the recent increase in peripheral nerve block practiced in developed countries is the greater proportion of surgical procedures carried out as 'day cases'. Regional anesthesia plays a fundamental role in the future of day case or ambulatory anesthesia, both as an intrinsic component of the anesthetic technique and for effective postoperative analgesia.[4] Currently, 60–70% of all surgical procedures performed in the USA are day cases. It is likely that peripheral nerve block, used appropriately in the ambulatory setting, decreases the time to discharge from hospital, improves patient satisfaction and postoperative analgesia, facilitates rehabilitation, and results in fewer complications than conventional analgesic techniques.

Third, the practice of peripheral nerve block has increased because of advances in technique, equipment, and our understanding of how and when it is indicated. These advances include the use of superior peripheral nerve stimulators and ultrasound for nerve localization and the use of indwelling catheters for 'continuous' techniques.

THE CONTENT

This publication comprises a textbook, atlas, and practical guide to peripheral nerve block, which presents material as text and images, including video clips, magnetic resonance (MR) images, still photographs, and line drawings. It is probably best regarded and used as an educational tool.

The textbook is in two parts. Part I covers the history, pharmacologic principles, and clinical applications of peripheral nerve blockade as well as the materials and equipment currently in use. In Part II, each chapter addresses a single block and describes its specific indications, relevant anatomy (including surface anatomy), and how the procedure is performed. The anatomy is presented using photographs of cadaveric dissections and volunteers (for surface anatomy), MR images, and sometimes line drawings. On the accompanying DVD-ROM, the anatomy and block technique are demonstrated using video clips; 'live' anatomy and spread of injectate are demonstrated using MR images. Chapters in Part II contain 'clinical pearls' intended to impart specific advice for improving success rates or avoiding problems. Associated with each chapter is a self-assessment section aimed at providing a means of evaluating both retention and comprehension of the information presented. This can be found at the associated website.

We have carefully selected the blocks for inclusion as those that are currently an established part of clinical anesthetic practice. We have attempted to describe those that will be of greatest interest and use to clinicians learning or practicing peripheral nerve blockade today. For instance, although para-sacral, subgluteal, popliteal, and other approaches have been described for block of the sciatic nerve, we have opted to describe only the more widely practiced classic anterior and posterior approaches. We have also excluded central neuraxial blocks (spinal and epidural techniques) and pediatric peripheral nerve blocks.

THE READERSHIP MOST LIKELY TO BENEFIT

It is widely recognized that anesthetists are incompletely trained unless they are proficient in the performance of peripheral nerve block.[5] Anesthetists comprise the single largest group of hospital doctors. Approximately 5% of all physicians in the USA practice anesthesia. In some countries, anesthesia is also practiced by nurse anesthetists.

The material contained in both the textbook and the DVD-ROM will be of greatest use to those practicing or learning anesthesia as a specialty. This group includes anesthetists (anesthesiologists), anesthetic trainees, and nurse anesthetists. Used in slightly different ways, this publication will provide a useful introduction to the practice of peripheral nerve blockade; a means of preparing for examinations (boards and fellow-ships); and a means of extending the range of practitioners' techniques or refreshing them with regard to a particular technique that they have not performed for some time. We have made no assumptions as to the background or experience of our readers. Therefore the techniques and practice are explained from first principles: anatomic, pharmacologic, and safety. Occasional practitioners of peripheral nerve blockade—whether anesthetists, emergency medicine physicians, or surgeons—are strongly advised to review Part I before moving to Part II to learn how to perform a particular block.

HOW TO USE THE CONTENT MOST EFFECTIVELY

First, it is important that readers who have little or no experience with peripheral nerve blocks—such as anesthetic trainees commencing the 'regional' or peripheral nerve block module of their training program—learn the principles underlying peripheral nerve blockade, outlined in Part I of the textbook, before studying specific blocks. This is intended to avoid the risk of training or being trained as a technician. It is essential that

peripheral nerve blocks be performed only by a practitioner with a sound understanding of how neural blockade is pharmacologically induced. This is to ensure that informed decisions are made regarding the suitability of a patient for peripheral nerve blockade or how best to treat a complication.

Second, an understanding of the anatomy (surface landmarks, nerves, plexuses, and their relations) relevant to a block is essential to ensure that a successful block is consistently and safely achieved. The anatomic material presented comprises text, line drawings, still photographs, video clips, and MR images. Our suggestion is that the relevant anatomy sections be read from the textbook with immediate reference to the accompanying still images in order to reinforce the conceptualization of the structures. This represents the first step to forming a mental image or model of the region. The second step entails playing the video clips of cadaveric dissection from the DVD-ROM and revising the still images, which are also displayed on the DVD-ROM for convenience. The next step in learning the relevant anatomy is to play the surface anatomy video clip, because this represents the bridge between the mental anatomic model that has been formed and the block technique, displayed immediately after the surface anatomy on each video clip.

Third, readers who wish to refresh their memory on a particular block, or commence learning about a new block, should first read the appropriate chapter in the textbook and then use the corresponding chapter in the DVD-ROM to reinforce (using video clips and MR images) the information they have read.

Fourth, it is advisable that the self-assessment sections be undertaken only after all the material on a particular block has been covered. The questions are designed to test both retention of information about and understanding of the relevant anatomy, technique, and clinical application of the block.

Finally, as readers may not be familiar with viewing MR images, a brief outline of the equipment used, principles, and image characteristics is presented below. This is worth reading before attempting to collate the MR images with either the cadaveric or surface anatomy images presented.

MAGNETIC RESONANCE IMAGING

Equipment

We use MR images in this textbook and DVD-ROM because of the excellent soft tissue contrast they provide, without exposing our volunteers to the ionizing radiation associated with computerized tomography and X-ray. Using the combination of a strong magnetic field and radiofrequency pulses, magnetic resonance imaging (MRI) obtains a digitized image of an anatomic area.

We used the Toshiba 0.35T OPART™, open system.[6] This scanner uses superconducting technology and high-speed gradients to produce high-quality images. The scanner was selected on the basis of its well-documented advantages; namely, that its open architecture allows comfortable volunteer positioning, easy access for injection, and prevents problems associated with claustrophobia.[7–9] A number of transmit and receive coils were used, appropriate to the anatomic area being scanned.

Physical principles

The images produced by MRI display contrast resolution between tissues due to the differences in their T1 recovery and T2 decay times. Tissues, at a subatomic level, are influenced by the magnetic field, which is both static and varying (gradients). Different tissues have different T1 recovery and T2 decay times due to differences in their precessional rates. Fat has a very short T1 time and water a long T1 time, such that fat displays as bright (high) signal and water displays as dark (low) signal in T1-weighted images. For T2 weighting, the time to echo must be long enough for the T2 decay times of fat and water to differentiate, and when this occurs, fat has a shorter T2 time than water.

In diagnostic MRI, contrast agents are used to enhance the contrast between normal tissue and pathology. This is more important on T1-weighted images, where water and tumors demonstrate similar low-signal intensities. The use of contrast agents selectively affects the T1 and T2 times of these tissues.[10] We used contrast to imitate and visualize the degree of spread of local anesthetic and to highlight anatomic structures.

Contrast agent

The contrast agent used is a gadolinium (Gd)-based agent; Gd is a paramagnetic material that has a positive effect on the local magnetic field. When it is near water, which has long T1 and T2 times, it causes a change in the local magnetic moment of the adjacent water molecules. This has the effect of reducing the T1 relaxation time of water, which allows water to give higher signal intensity on T1-weighted images. Thus Gd and other paramagnetic substances are known as T1 enhancement agents.[11]

As a free ion, Gd is quite toxic and has a biological half-life of several weeks, the kidneys and liver demonstrating greatest uptake. For this reason, Gd is aligned with a substance known as a chelate. The chelate works by attaching to eight of the nine free-binding sites of the Gd molecule. This reduces Gd's toxic effect because it facilitates faster excretion. The contrast agent that we used was gadopentetate dimeglumine (Magnevist®), which has the Gd molecule attached to a chelate called diethylenetriaminepenta-acetic acid (DTPA). This produces the complex molecule Gd-DTPA and is a relatively safe, water-soluble contrast agent. However, the addition of a chelate affects the ability of the Gd to reduce the T1 recovery time of the adjacent tissue. Thus the use of a chelate must take into consideration the rate of uptake of the Gd-DTPA agent, the relative T1 recovery time of the tissue, and the safety of the complex.[12] The contrast was diluted to 1:250 in order to obtain the best signal. This level of dilution was selected following serial testing (on 'phantoms') using different degrees of dilution.

Image characteristics

There are a number of different sequences available to MRI scanners. We used T1-weighted spin echo sequences primarily, supplemented by fat-saturated sequences. T1-weighted MR images show very good soft-tissue contrast and also show enhancement from Gd-based contrast agents. As explained, due to differing relaxation times of fat and water on T1-weighted tissues, fat displays as high signal (bright) and water displays as low signal (dark).[10] In the images where contrast is displayed, the short relaxation time of the Gd-based contrast agent enables the contrast to have high signal. On some images, the high signal of both fat and contrast may be similar, but by comparing with precontrast images and fat-saturated images it is possible to differentiate between the signals.

A number of sequences were performed for each region. In some instances, image windowing and magnification were performed in order to clearly demonstrate the structures. The images that best illustrate the anatomy and contrast spread were selected for inclusion in the atlas. As in many clinical MR images, motion artifact is detectable in some images. These have only been included if the image has educational value despite the artifact.

References

1. Hadzic A, Vloka JD, Kuroda MM, et al. The practice of peripheral nerve blocks in the United States: a national survey. Reg Anesth Pain Med 1998; 23: 241–246.
2. Mingus ML. Recovery advantages of regional compared with general anesthesia: adult patients. J Clin Anesth 1995; 7: 628–633.
3. Chelly JE, Greger J, Gebhard R, et al. Continuous femoral nerve blocks improve recovery and outcome of patients undergoing total knee arthroplasty. Arthroplasty 2001; 16: 436–445.
4. White PF, Smith I. Ambulatory anesthesia: past, present and future. Int Anesthesiol Clin 1994; 32: 1–16.
5. Kopacz DJ, Bridenbaugh CD. Are anesthetic residencies failing regional anesthesia? Reg Anesth 1993; 18: 84–87.
6. Toshiba Corp. MRI system, OPART, product information. Toshiba Corp.; 1998.
7. Dworkin JS. Open field magnetic resonance imaging; system and environment. The technology and potential of open magnetic resonance imaging. Berlin: Springer-Verlag; 2000: 45–56.
8. Kaufman L, Carlson J, Li A, et al. Open-magnet technology for magnetic resonance imaging. In: Open field magnetic resonance imaging: equipment, diagnosis and interventional procedures. Berlin: Springer-Verlag; 2000: 25–30.

9. Spouse E, Gedroyc WM. MRI of the claustrophobic patient: interventionally configured magnets. Br J Radiol 2000; 73: 146–151.

10. Westbrook C, Kaut C. MRI in practice. 2nd edn. Oxford: Blackwell Science; 1998: 252–258.

11. Muroff L. MRI contrast: current agents and issues. Appl Radiol 2001; 30(8): 8–14.

12. Runge V. The safety of MR contrast media: a literature review. Appl Radiol 2001; 30(8): 5–7.

CHAPTER 2

Regional anesthesia in perspective: history, current role, and the future

The *doctrine of specific energies of the senses*, proclaimed by Johannes P. Mueller (1801–58) in 1826—that it is the nerves that determine what the mind perceives—opened up a new field of scientific thought and research into nerve function.[1] This led directly to the theory that pain is a separate and distinct sense, formulated by Moritz S. Schiff (1823–96) in 1858.[2] Yet by 1845, Sir Francis Rynd (1801–61) had already delivered a morphine solution to a nerve for the purpose of relieving intractable neuralgia (Box 2.1).[3] This appears to be the first documented nerve block as we understand the term today. Rynd, however, delivered his solution by means of gravity through a cannula. The first use of a syringe and hypodermic needle was not recorded until 10 years later, in 1855, by Alexander Wood (1817–84) in Edinburgh.[4] Wood used a graduated glass syringe and needle to achieve the same end as Rynd.

Box 2.1 Medical history: the first hypodermic injection

18th May 1844

She thought the eye was being torn out of her head, and her cheek from her face; it lasted about two hours, and then suddenly disappeared on taking a mouthful of ice. She had not had a return for three months, when it came back even worse than before, quite suddenly, one night on going out of a warm room into the cold air. On this attack she was seized with chilliness, shivering, and slight nausea; the left eye lacrimated profusely, and became red with pain; it went in darts through her whole head, face, and mouth, and the paroxysm lasted for three weeks, during which time she never slept. She was bled and blistered, and took opium for it, but without relief. It continued coming at irregular intervals, but each time more intense in character, until at last, weary of her existence, she came to Dublin for relief.

On the 3rd of June a solution of fifteen grains of acetate of morphia, dissolved in one drachm of creosote, was introduced to the supra-orbital nerve, and along the course of the temporal, malar, and buccal nerves, by four punctures of an instrument made for the purpose. In the space of a minute all pain (except that caused by the operation, which was very slight) had ceased, and she slept better that night than she had for months. After an interval of a week she had a slight return of pain in the gums of both upper and under jaw. The fluid was again introduced by two punctures made in the gum of each jaw, and the pain disappeared.

Francis Rynd (1801–61)

FRCSI 1830; appointed Surgeon to the Meath Hospital 1836

(From Rynd 1845.[3])

Carl Koller (1857–1944) was an intern at the Ophthalmologic Clinic at the University of Vienna in 1884. He was searching for a topical local anesthetic and, on the advice of Sigmund Freud (1856–1939), studied cocaine. Following self-experimentation, Koller performed an operation for glaucoma under topical anesthesia on September 11, 1884. He immediately wrote a paper for the Congress of Ophthalmology (held on September 15 of that year) which was published soon after in the *Lancet*.[5] The remarkable effectiveness of cocaine as an anesthetic agent led to its immediate widespread use in this area.[6,7]

In the same year as Koller's achievement, 1884, William Stewart Halsted (1852–1922) performed the first documented brachial plexus anesthetic under direct vision at Johns Hopkins,[8] although it was 1911 before Hirschel and Kulenkampff performed the first percutaneous axillary and supraclavicular brachial plexus blocks.[9,10] By the 1890s, Carl Ludwig Schleich (1859–1922) in Germany and Paul Reclus (1847–1914) in France were seriously writing on the subject of infiltration anesthesia, first with water and later with weak solutions of cocaine.[11,12]

Anesthesia as a specialty had not yet developed at this stage, because the surgeon infiltrated as he operated. Victor Pauchet (1869–1936) was the first to point out a new technique of *regional anesthesia* in which the procedure was carried out by an assistant in advance. In his 1914 textbook *L'Anesthésie Régionale*, the first of its kind, he stated that he had witnessed Reclus's technique at first hand 25 years before, and now wished to emphasize the novel concept of regional anesthesia and the emergence of anesthesia or anesthesiology as a specialty.[13]

Sydney Ormond Goldan (1869–1944), describing himself as an anesthetist, had published the first anesthesia chart in 1900.[14] It was designed for monitoring the course of 'intraspinal cocainization' and helped lay the foundation for the careful record-keeping that is a cornerstone of modern anesthesia.

Gaston Labat (1876–1934) worked and trained under Pauchet in France in 1917–18.[15] He learned much from treating the casualties of World War I, and in 1922 published the first edition of *Regional Anesthesia: Techniques and Clinical Applications*, one of the first English-language texts on the subject.[16] Many of his illustrations and techniques continue to have relevance today.

On September 29, 1920, Labat arrived at the Mayo Clinic, Rochester, Minnesota, to teach regional anesthesia to the clinic's surgeons. From his brief 9-month period there and following tenure at Bellevue Hospital, New York University, he was to have a major influence on the development of the specialty of anesthesia in the USA.[17] His influence on practitioners such as John Lundy, Ralph Waters, and Emory Rovenstine—pioneers in the development of the specialty—was substantial and the American Society of Regional Anesthesia was initially to have been named after him.[18]

The American Board of Anesthesiology was formed in 1938 and held its first written examinations in March 1939. Here, Labat's legacy continued. In the anatomy section all five questions related to regional anesthesia blocks; two of the five pharmacology questions dealt with local anesthetics in regional anesthesia; and one of the pathology questions dealt with regional anesthesia.[19]

Developments continued in the subspecialty through the twentieth century (see Box 2.2) to the point where in 1980 a survey of American anesthesiology residency programs reported the use of regional anesthesia in 21.3% of cases, in 1990 in 29.8% of cases, and in 2000 in 30.2% of cases.[20–22] The majority of these cases, however, involve obstetric anesthesia or pain medicine, which has raised concern in some quarters as to the future place of peripheral nerve blockade in perioperative anesthetic practice. This future, indeed, may lie in the areas of acute pain management and patient satisfaction.

Continuous peripheral nerve blocks using catheters have been in use since 1946.[23] They have been shown to provide

---

Box 2.2 Development of regional anesthesia

1826	Mueller: doctrine of specific energies of the senses
1845	Rynd: first nerve block
1855	Wood: needle and syringe
1858	Schiff: pain defined as a specific sense
1884	Koller: cocaine used for topical anesthesia
	Halsted: first brachial plexus block
1890	Schleich & Reclus: infiltration anesthesia
1900	Goldan: anesthesia charts
1911	Hirschel & Kulenkampff: percutaneous brachial plexus block
	Stoffel: galvanic current applied to nerve
1914	Pauchet: *L'Anésthesie Régionale*
1922	Labat: *Regional Anesthesia: Techniques and Clinical Applications*
1923	American Society of Regional Anesthesia founded
1930	Labat: posterior approach to the stellate ganglion
1939	Rovenstine & Wertheim: cervical plexus block
1940	Patrick: current supraclavicular brachial plexus technique
1946	Ansboro: continuous brachial plexus block
1954	Moore: paratracheal approach to stellate ganglion
1958	Burnham: axillary brachial plexus perivascular technique
1964	Winnie & Collins: subclavian brachial plexus block
1970	Winnie: interscalene brachial plexus block
1973	Montgomery, Raj: nerve stimulator in contemporary practice
1993	Collum, Courtney: lateral popliteal approach to the sciatic nerve
1995	Kilka: vertical infraclavicular brachial plexus block

effective postoperative analgesia, be opioid-sparing, and result in improved rehabilitation and high patient satisfaction.[24–26] With refining of the techniques over the intervening half-century, a number of clinicians have used them with great effectiveness. To date, however, their use has been largely confined to inpatients because worries about motor weakness, patient injury, catheter migration, and local anesthetic toxicity have persisted. Concurrently, up to 70 or 80% of patients complain of severe pain following ambulatory surgery, requiring continued opioid medication for up to a week in many cases.[27,28]

In the early 2000s, a number of authors reported the use of continuous peripheral nerve catheters in the ambulatory setting with a high degree of success, few complications, and good levels of patient acceptance and satisfaction.[29–32] As these techniques are still in their infancy, a number of special precautions were taken in these studies to ensure safety in the home environment. In addition, as the early pioneers had to defend their practice, it is certain these new pioneers will have to do likewise with these new developments. Further research will likely define the indications and limitations of this technology.

Long-acting peripheral nerve block has been used with a high degree of efficacy, safety, and satisfaction in the ambulatory setting, and is practiced by many regional anesthetists.[33,34] Single-injection extended-duration (72-h) local anesthetic agents have been heralded for many years.[35] When, and if, they become a reality we may see a rapid expansion in the use of regional anesthetic techniques as well as the resurrection of the original infiltration techniques as practiced by Schleich and Reclus.

The concept of patient satisfaction has been often dismissed as a parameter too difficult to measure. Unfortunately, the lack of an accepted model of patient satisfaction has hindered progress.[36] In recent years, however, a few authors have described the development of global measurement tools and psychometrically constructed questionnaires that produce reliable results; these tools have been applied prospectively in large patient populations.[37,38] Parameters such as improved pain relief and reduced postoperative nausea and vomiting are some of the factors influenced positively by regional anesthesia, and these are also indicators of high patient satisfaction. It can be said that patient satisfaction has become an important indicator of quality of medical care and an important endpoint in outcomes research.[39]

References

1. Riese W, Arrington GE Jr. The history of Johannes Muller's doctrine of the specific energies of the senses: original and later versions. Bull Hist Med 1963; 37: 179–183.
2. Dallenbach KM. Pain: history and present status. Am J Psychol 1939; 52: 331.
3. Rynd F. Neuralgia—introduction of fluid to the nerve. Dublin Med Press 1845; 13: 167–168.
4. Wood A. New method of treating neuralgia by the direct application of opiates to the painful points. Edinb Med Surg J 1855; 82: 265–281.
5. Koller C. On the use of cocaine for producing anaesthesia on the eye. Lancet 1884; 2: 990–992.
6. Hepburn NJ. Some notes on hydrochlorate of cocaine. Med Rec (NY) 1884; 26: 534.
7. Bull CS. The hydrochlorate of cocaine as a local anaesthetic in ophthalmic surgery. NY Med J 1884; 40: 609–612.
8. Halsted WS. Surgical papers. Baltimore: Johns Hopkins Press; 1925: 167.
9. Hirschel G. Anaesthesia of the brachial plexus for operations on the upper extremity. Med Wochenschr 1911; 5: 1555–1960.
10. Kulenkampff D. Die Anasthesia des plexus brachialis. Zentralbl Chir 1911; 38: 1337.
11. Schleich CL. Zur Infiltrations anasthesie. Therapeutisch Monatshefte 1894; 8: 429.
12. Reclus P. Analgésie locale par la cocaine. Rev Chir 1889; 9: 913–916.
13. Pauchet V, Sourdat P. L'Anésthesie Régionale. Paris: Octave Doin et Fils, Editeurs; 1914.
14. Goldan SO. Intraspinal cocainization for surgical anaesthesia. Phila Med J 1900; 6: 850–853.
15. Brown DL, Winnie AP. Biography of Louis Gaston Labat, MD. Reg Anesth 1992; 22: 218–222.
16. Labat G. Regional anesthesia: techniques and clinical applications. Philadelphia: WB Saunders; 1922.
17. Bacon RD, Gaston Labat, John Lundy, Emery Rovenstine, and the Mayo Clinic. The spread of regional anesthesia in America between the World Wars. J Clin Anesth 2002; 14: 315–320.
18. Betcher AM, Ciliberti PM, Wood PM, et al. The jubilee year of organized anesthesia. Anesthesiology 1956; 17: 226–264.
19. Bacon DR, Darwish H, Emory A. To define a specialty: a brief history of the American Board of Anesthesiology's first written examination. J Clin Anesth 1992; 4: 489–497.
20. Bridenbaugh L. Are anesthesia resident programs failing regional anesthesia? Reg Anesth 1982; 7: 26–28.
21. Kopacz DJ, Bridenbaugh LD. Are anesthesia residency programs failing regional anesthesia? The past, present, and future. Reg Anesth 1993; 18: 84–87.
22. Kopacz DJ, Neal JM. Regional anesthesia and pain medicine: residency training—the year 2000. Reg Anesth Pain Med 2002; 27: 9–14.
23. Ansboro F. Method of continuous brachial plexus block. Am J Surg 1946; 71: 716–722.
24. Selander D. Catheter technique in axillary plexus block. Acta Anaesth Scand 1977; 21: 324–329.
25. Dahl J, Christiansen C, Daugaard J, et al. Continuous blockade of the lumbar plexus after knee surgery—postoperative analgesia and bupivacaine plasma concentrations. A controlled clinical trial. Anaesthesia 1988; 43: 1015–1018.
26. Capdevila X, Barthelet Y, Biboulet P, et al. Effects of perioperative analgesic technique on the surgical outcome and duration of rehabilitation after major knee surgery. Anesthesiology 1999; 91: 8–15.
27. Chung F, Mezei G. Adverse outcomes in ambulatory anesthesia. Can J Anesth 1999; 46: R18–R26.
28. McHugh GA, Thoms GMM. The management of pain following day-case surgery. Anaesthesia 2002; 57: 270–275.
29. Ilfeld B, Morey T, Enneking F. Continuous infraclavicular block for postoperative pain control at home: a randomized double-blind placebo-controlled study. Anesthesiology 2002; 96: 1297–1304.
30. Ilfeld BM, Morey TE, Wang DR, et al. Continuous popliteal sciatic nerve block for postoperative pain control at home: a randomized,

double-blinded, placebo-controlled study. Anesthesiology 2002; 97: 959–965.

31. Rawal N, Allvin R, Axelsson K, et al. Patient-controlled regional analgesia (PCRA) at home. Controlled comparison between bupivacaine and ropivacaine brachial plexus analgesia. Anesthesiology 2002; 96: 1290–1296.

32. Grant SA, Nielsen KC, Greengrass RA, et al. Continuous peripheral nerve block for ambulatory surgery. Reg Anesth Pain Med 2001; 26: 209–214.

33. Klein SM, Nielsen KC, Greengrass RA, et al. Ambulatory discharge after long-acting peripheral nerve blockade: 2382 blocks with ropivacaine. Anesth Analg 2002; 94: 65–70.

34. Klein SM, Pietrobon R, Nielsen KC, et al. Peripheral nerve blockade with long-acting local anesthetics: a survey of the society for ambulatory anesthesia. Anesth Analg 2002; 94: 71–76.

35. Klein SM. Beyond the hospital: continuous peripheral nerve blocks at home [editorial]. Anesthesiology 2002; 96: 1283–1285.

36. Wu CL, Naqibuddin M, Fleischer LA. Measurement of patient satisfaction as an outcome of regional anesthesia and analgesia: a systematic review. Reg Anesth Pain Med 2001; 26: 196–208.

37. Myles PS, Williams DL, Hendrata M, et al. Patient satisfaction after anaesthesia and surgery: results of a prospective study of 10,811 patients. Br J Anaesth 2000; 84: 6–10.

38. Tong D, Chung F, Wong D. Predictive factors in global and anesthesia satisfaction in ambulatory surgical patients. Anesthesiology 1997; 87: 856–864.

39. Schug SA. Patient satisfaction—politically correct fashion of the nineties or a valuable measure of outcome? Reg Anesth Pain Med 2001; 26: 193–195.

CHAPTER 3

Local anesthetics

THE PERIPHERAL NERVE

Applied anatomy

The typical nerve cell has been traditionally described in terms of having a cell body (perikaryon), multiple dendrites, and a single axon (Fig. 3.1). Sensory neurons are classified as unipolar; that is, they have an axon that divides to extend a branch to both the spinal cord and the periphery. Motor neurons are classified as multipolar because, in addition to an axon, they possess many dendrites. Impulses arriving via the dendrites and cell body are integrated at the axon hillock, a specialized area of the cell body. Summation of excitatory and inhibitory impulses occurs at the axon hillock and determines whether impulses are generated or not.

The axon is always enclosed within a nutriprotective Schwann cell envelope. Most are further invested in a myelin sheath formed by a single Schwann cell wrapped many times around the axon and interrupted periodically at the nodes of Ranvier. Many unmyelinated nerves, on the other hand, may have their axons enclosed within the folds of a single Schwann cell (Fig. 3.2).

The nerve cell membrane, in common with all cells of the body, comprises a phospholipid bilayer traversed by proteins that selectively regulate the influx and efflux of ions and molecules, act as hormone and transmitter receptors, are involved in cell-to-cell interactions, and enhance the structural integrity of the membrane (Fig. 3.3). It is the specialized nature of some of these proteins that is responsible for the unique character of nerve cells.[2]

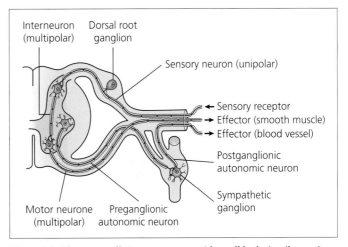

Figure 3.1 The nerve cell. Sensory neuron with a cell body (perikaryon) and an axon with long peripheral and short central branches (unipolar nerve cell); interneuron with numerous dendrites, a cell body, and one short axon (multipolar nerve cell); motor neuron with a great many dendrites, a cell body, and a long peripheral axon (multipolar). (From Strichatz GR. Neural Physiology and Local Anesthetic Action. In Cousins MJ, Bridenbaugh PO (eds). Neural Blockade in Clinical Anesthesia and Management of Pain, 3rd edn. Philadelphia: © Lippincott-Raven; 1998.)

Ionic basis of conduction

A special membrane protein, the Na^+–K^+ ATPase pump, is responsible for the transmembrane concentration gradient of these ions peculiar to nerve cells. It transports sodium out of the cell and potassium into it.[3] At rest, the membrane is selectively permeable to K^+, resulting in an efflux of positive

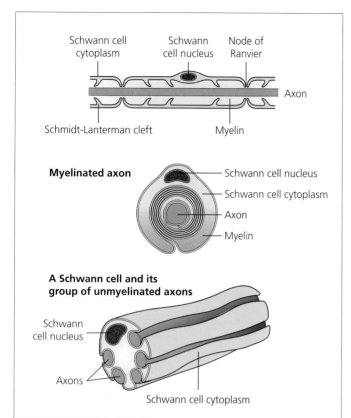

Figure 3.2 The axon. Myelinated axon in longitudinal section (**A**), showing the relation of the myelin sheath to the nodes of Ranvier, and transverse section (**B**), showing how the Schwann cell wraps around one axon many times to form the multiple layers of the myelin sheath. A Schwann cell and its group of unmyelinated axons (**C**); many unmyelinated axons are embedded in the folds of a single Schwann cell.
(From Strichatz GR. Neural Physiology and Local Anesthetic Action. In Cousins MJ, Bridenbaugh PO (eds). Neural Blockade in Clinical Anesthesia and Management of Pain, 3rd edn. Philadelphia: © Lippincott-Raven; 1998.)

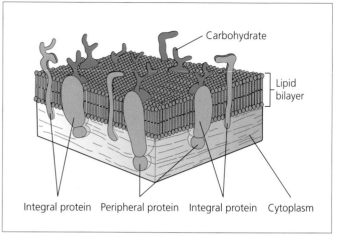

Figure 3.3 The axonal membrane. A phospholipid bilayer traversed by proteins. Carbohydrate molecules attached to proteins and lipids on the extracellular surface of the membrane form a 'cell coat'. The lipid bilayer consists of densely packed phospholipids. Integral proteins and peripheral proteins only on the cytoplasmic surface are associated with enzymatic and receptor functions.
(From Strichatz GR. Neural Physiology and Local Anesthetic Action. In Cousins MJ, Bridenbaugh PO (eds). Neural Blockade in Clinical Anesthesia and Management of Pain, 3rd edn. Philadelphia: © Lippincott-Raven; 1998.)

charge. Thus the interior of the cell is negatively charged relative to the exterior; this resting membrane potential is in the order of -70–80 mV. Because of its chemical and electrical gradient, there is a tendency for Na^+ to enter the cell.

Temporal and spatial summation of excitatory and inhibitory potentials occurs at the axon hillock. Small net depolarizations of 15–20 mV will raise the membrane potential to -55 mV, resulting in a voltage-dependent opening of Na^+ channels and a rapid change in transmembrane potential to $+40$ mV.[4–6] This is shortly followed by the opening of K^+ channels, and the subsequent outward flow of K^+ returns the membrane potential to normal and beyond (the refractory period where it is more difficult to stimulate the nerve).[3] The Na^+–K^+ pump then serves to restore the chemical gradient to its initial state. These changes in transmembrane potential account for the familiar action potential (Fig. 3.4). The electrical changes occurring during the action potential serve to open adjacent voltage-dependent Na^+ channels, and so the action potential is propagated along the axon. Because the area immediately preceding the action potential is in the refractory period, the action potential is propagated in one direction only.

STRUCTURE AND FUNCTION OF LOCAL ANESTHETICS

Local anesthetics consist of a lipophilic aromatic ring connected by a hydrocarbon chain to a hydrophilic tertiary amine (Fig. 3.5). The lipophilic moiety is responsible for the anesthetic activity of the molecule. The drugs are classified as amide or ester local anesthetics based on the nature of the bond linking the hydrocarbon chain and the aromatic ring. The ester drugs are rapidly hydrolyzed by plasma and other esterases,[8–12] and have been associated with allergic and hypersensitivity reactions linked to their breakdown product *para*-aminobenzoic acid.[13] In contrast, amides are relatively stable compounds, are metabolized in the liver, and allergic reactions to them are exceedingly rare. The comparative pharmacology of local anesthetics is shown in Table 3.1.

Local anesthetics produce conduction blockade through reversible inhibition of Na^+ channel function.[15,16] Physiological studies have demonstrated that local anesthetics inhibit stimulated channels more readily than resting channels; this is known as phasic block and tonic block, respectively.[17] The modulated receptor hypothesis has been proposed to explain these features.[18,19] It is based on the fact that Na^+ channels pass

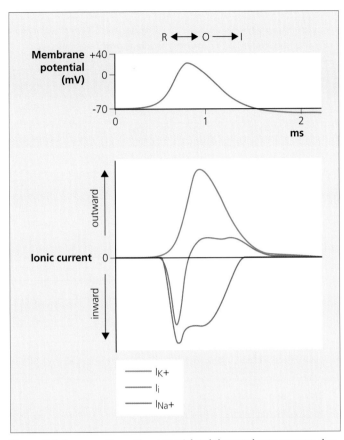

Figure 3.4 A propagating action potential and the membrane currents that produce it. See text for details. I_{K+}, outward K^+ current; I_{Na+}, inward Na^+ current; I_i, net ionic current across the membrane.
(From Strichatz GR. Neural Physiology and Local Anesthetic Action. In Cousins MJ, Bridenbaugh PO (eds). Neural Blockade in Clinical Anesthesia and Management of Pain, 3rd edn. Philadelphia: © Lippincott-Raven; 1998.)

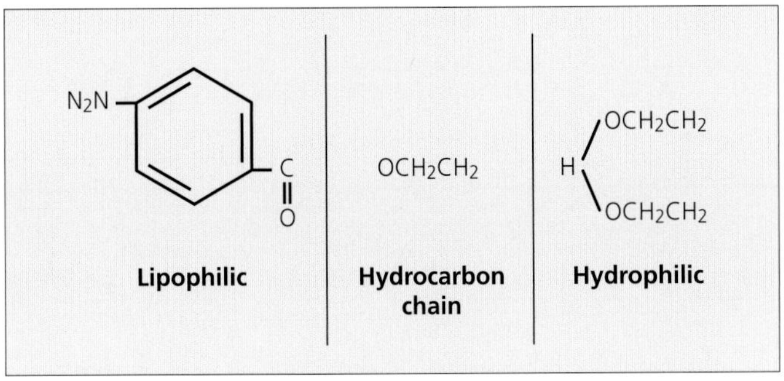

Figure 3.5 Structure of local anesthetics. Local anesthetics comprise a lipophilic and a hydrophilic portion separated by a connecting hydrocarbon chain.
(From Stoelting RK. Pharmacology and physiology in anesthetic practice. 2nd edn. Philadelphia: © JB Lippincott; 1991.)

through various states during membrane depolarization. They begin in the resting state (R), pass through an intermediate closed form (C), to reach an open form (O), and then close to reach an inactivated state (I). According to the modulated receptor hypothesis, local anesthetics have greater affinity for Na^+ channels in the O and I configurations than in the C and R configurations. Thus local anesthetics will more readily bind Na^+ channels of stimulated or active nerves.

Two possible binding sites for local anesthetics have been identified on the Na^+ channel.[15,18] The first site is thought to be responsible for phasic block and is situated near the channel pore. Binding and unbinding from this site is relatively slow. The second site is on the inner aspect of the channel in the hydrophobic center of the membrane. Binding and dissociation at this site is rapid.

PHARMACODYNAMICS

Local anesthetics are poorly water-soluble bases and are therefore prepared as hydrochloride salts. The ionized and non-ionized forms of local anesthetics exist in equilibrium:

$$B + H^+ \rightleftharpoons BH^+$$

Their ratio is given by the Henderson–Hasselbach equation:

$$pKa = pH - [B].[BH^+]$$

Both the ionized and non-ionized forms can inhibit Na^+ channels.[20–23] The observations that tertiary amine local anesthetics are more potent when applied externally at an alkaline pH, or applied directly internally, suggest that the neutral form of the local anesthetic traverses the membrane, where it assumes its ionized form once again to become active at the internal aspect of the Na^+ channel.[24] Following injection, the alkaline pH of the tissues releases the base:

$$B.HCl + HCO_3^- \rightleftharpoons B + H_2CO_3 + Cl^-$$

Physiochemical properties of local anesthetics

Ionization

The degree of ionization depends on the pKa of the agent. The pKa is defined as the negative logarithm of the dissociation constant (Ka) of the conjugate acid. It is equal to the pH at which the local anesthetic is 50% ionized. The greater the pKa of the base, the smaller the proportion existing in its non-ionized form at any pH, and so the slower the speed of onset.[25,26]

Lipid solubility

The lipid solubility of local anesthetics may be expressed in terms of their water:oil partition coefficient. A high coefficient indicates a high degree of lipid solubility and ready penetration of nerve fibers. While balanced by the high fraction of drug

Classification	Potency	Onset	Duration after infiltration (min)	Maximum single dose for infiltration (adult, mg)*
Esters				
Procaine	1	Slow	45–60	500
Chloroprocaine	4	Rapid	30–45	600
Tetracaine	16	Slow	60–180	100 (topical)
Amides				
Lidocaine	1	Rapid	60–120	300
Mepivacaine	1	Slow	90–180	300
Bupivacaine	4	Slow	240–480	175
Etidocaine	4	Slow	240–480	300
Prilocaine	1	Slow	60–120	400
Ropivacaine†	–	–	–	–

Classification	Toxic plasma concentration (μg/ml)	pK	Fraction nonionized (%) pH 7.2	pH 7.4	pH 7.6	Protein binding (%)
Esters						
Procaine	–	8.9	2	3	5	6
Chloroprocaine	–	8.7	3	5	7	–
Tetracaine	–	8.5	5	7	11	76
Amides						
Lidocaine	> 5	7.9	17	25	33	70
Mepivacaine	> 5	7.6	28	39	50	77
Bupivacaine	~ 1.5	8.1	11	15	24	95
Etidocaine	~ 2	7.7	24	33	44	94
Prilocaine	> 5	7.9	17	24	33	55
Ropivacaine†	> 4	8.1	–	–	94	–

Classification	Lipid solubility	Volume of distribution (L)	Clearance (L/min)	Elimination half-time (min)
Esters				
Procaine	0.6	–	–	–
Chloroprocaine	–	–	–	–
Tetracaine	80	–	–	–
Amides				
Lidocaine	2.9	91	0.95	96
Mepivacaine	1.0	84	9.78	114
Bupivacaine	28	73	0.47	210
Etidocaine	141	133	1.22	156
Prilocaine	0.9	–	–	–
Ropivacaine†	–	–	–	–

*Use only as a guideline; dose may be increased if solution contains epinephrine.
†Resembles bupivacaine
(From Covino & Vassallo 1976,[14] with permission of Grune and Stratton.)

Table 3.1. Comparative pharmacology of local anesthetics

that is therefore in the non-ionized state, in general, high lipid solubility is associated with increased potency and duration of effect.[26,27]

Protein binding

The duration of action of local anesthetics is related to their degree of protein binding. The bound fraction constitutes a functional reservoir that is released as the free drug is distributed or eliminated. Because it is only the unbound fraction of drug that is active, a high degree of protein binding will also result in a slower onset rate.[28]

PHARMACOKINETICS

Local distribution

The local distribution of local anesthetics is affected by the physiochemical properties of the agent; the site of injection; the volume, mass, and concentration injected; and the presence or absence of vasoconstrictor substances.

The mass movement or bulk flow of an agent is a physical process and as such depends on the volume of drug injected, the rate of injection, and the physical barrier of the surrounding fibrous and fatty tissue.

Fick's Law explains the relations between the various factors affecting diffusion of a substance through a membrane:

$$dQ/dT = D.A.K.\Delta C/\delta$$

where dQ/dT is the rate of passive diffusion; D the diffusion coefficient of the drug in the membrane; A the area of the membrane; K the aqueous membrane partition coefficient of the drug; ΔC the concentration gradient; and δ the thickness of the membrane.

Local clearance of drug depends on the vascularity of the injection site and the degree of tissue binding. Therefore a rich capillary bed and little surrounding fatty tissue coupled with a low water:oil partition coefficient favors systemic absorption. The rate of absorption and hence initial plasma concentrations as a function of site of injection, vary as follows: spinal < plexus block < epidural < caudal < intercostal < intrapleural (Fig. 3.6).

Following absorption into the systemic circulation, local anesthetics are subjected to substantial sequestration by the lungs.[30,31] This is because of a high lung:blood partition coefficient and ion trapping of drug secondary to the low extravascular pH of the lungs. The drugs also bind plasma proteins, showing high affinity and low capacity for alpha$_1$-acid glycoprotein, and low affinity and high capacity for albumin. This binding is increased in the presence of cancer, trauma, chronic pain, and inflammatory disease, as well as in the postoperative period; it is significantly decreased in neonates because of their low plasma concentrations of alpha$_1$-

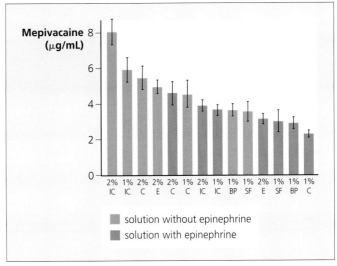

Figure 3.6 Systemic absorption of mepivacaine in humans after various regional block procedures as indicated by mean (±SEM) maximum plasma drug concentrations. IC, intercostal block; C, caudal block; E, epidural block; BP, brachial plexus block; SF, sciatic or femoral block; w/o, solution without epinephrine; w, with epinephrine. 1:200 000 (shaded). (From Tucker et al 1972,[29] with permission.)

acid glycoprotein. Further binding of drug takes place in the tissues. The long-acting group of amide local anesthetics are bound in plasma and tissue to a greater extent than the short-acting ones.[32–37]

The distribution of local anesthetics obeys the laws governing a three-compartment model of distribution and elimination. This can be described by:

- a distribution half-life, corresponding to the distribution of drug in tissues rich in blood supply;
- a transfer half-life, corresponding to the distribution in poorly vascularized tissues; and
- an elimination half-life, corresponding to the time necessary to eliminate 50% of the administered dose.

The volume of distribution in a steady state (VD$_{ss}$) is based on unbound plasma concentrations and reflects net tissue binding.

The half-life of elimination can be calculated following the intravenous injection of a bolus of drug. It allows one to anticipate the risk of drug accumulation in case of reinjection. For example, lidocaine has an elimination half-life of 96 min and bupivacaine 210 min.[14] Therefore as a rough guide one may readminister half the initial dose 1.5 and 3.5 h following the first injection, and in this way avoid drug accumulation.

Metabolism and excretion

Amide local anesthetics are metabolized in the liver and their elimination depends on their hepatic clearance. They can be divided into two groups depending on whether their hepatic extraction ratio is high (e.g. lidocaine, > 50%) or low (e.g. bupivacaine, < 40%). Those drugs with a high ratio have, therefore, perfusion-dependent clearance; those with a low ratio are subject to induction and inhibition of hepatic enzyme systems.[38]

As stated above, the ester drugs are rapidly hydrolyzed by plasma and other esterases, limiting their potential for toxicity.[8,9,11,39,40] Renal excretion of local anesthetics is of little importance, accounting for less than 6% of the dose. This may be increased, however, to 20% following acidification of the urine.[41]

NERVE BLOCK IN CLINICAL PRACTICE

Nerve fibers

Nerve fibers have been categorized into A, B, and C fibers. A fibers have been further divided into α, β, γ, and δ fibers. The important features of each category of nerve fiber are outlined in Table 3.2. A fibers are myelinated somatic nerves, B fibers myelinated preganglionic autonomic nerves, and C fibers unmyelinated nerves. The susceptibility of nerves to local anesthetics, in general, depends on their caliber, degree of myelination, and speed of conduction. However, as outlined below, further factors also come into play.

Minimum blocking concentration

The minimum blocking concentration (C_m) is the lowest concentration of a local anesthetic agent that will block conduction in a nerve in vitro. In vivo, the drug is injected in and about nerve trunks, fibrous sheaths, fatty tissue, and blood vessels. Therefore before reaching a nerve, it is subject to dilu-

tion, dispersion, fixation, destruction, and systemic absorption. Under these conditions, the minimum concentration necessary to block a nerve is much greater than the C_m. Consequently, lidocaine 1% is necessary to block a mixed somatic nerve that has a C_m for lidocaine of approximately 0.07%.[42]

Differential nerve block

Within a single peripheral nerve, one may observe complete block of pain fibers (Aδ and C) while motor and touch (Aα and Aβ) are spared. This is known as differential nerve block. A number of possible explanations for this phenomenon have been postulated. First, the time taken for a drug to diffuse into and along the course of a nerve, and so affect various fibers, may result in the clinical features observed. Second, the presence or absence of a myelin sheath may affect local anesthetic activity and penetration. Third, not all axons have the same sensitivity to local anesthetic agents because of variations in Na$^+$ channel and membrane lipid content.[43,44]

Nerve penetration

Peripheral nerves are organized so that the fibers innervating the distal portions of a limb are in the center of the nerve trunk and the more proximal structures are supplied from the outer layers of the trunk. Following deposition of the drug, one may therefore observe anesthesia of the more proximal limb structures before the distal ones (Fig. 3.7).

Regression of block is primarily dependent on diffusion from the nerve and absorption into the local vasculature. Drugs with high lipophilic solubility diffuse slowly from local tissues for reasons stated earlier, while the addition of adrenaline to local anesthetics results in local vasoconstriction and an increase of up to 50% in block duration.[46–48]

	Aα	Aβ	Aγ	Aδ	B	C
Diameter (μm)	12–20	5–12	5–12	1–4	1–3	0.5–1
Conduction speed	70–120	30–70	30–70	12–30	14.8	1.2
Myelination	+++	++	++	+	+	−
Function	Motor	Pressure, touch	Proprioception	Pain, temperature	Vasoconstriction	Pain, temperature
Onset of block	5th	4th	3rd	2nd	1st	2nd

(From Strichatz GR. Neural Physiology and Local Anesthetic Action. In Cousins MJ, Bridenbaugh PO (eds). Neural Blockade in Clinical Anesthesia and Management of Pain, 3rd edn. Philadelphia: © Lippincott-Raven; 1998.)

Table 3.2. Characteristics of different categories of nerve fiber

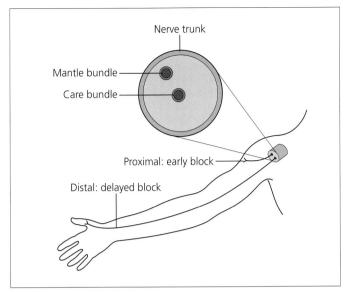

Figure 3.7 Somatopic distribution in peripheral nerve. Axons in large nerve trunks are arranged so that the outer fibers innervate the more proximal structures. The inner fibers innervate the more distal parts of a limb. (From de Jong RH. Physiology and pharmacology of local anesthesia. Springfield, IL, 1970. Courtesy of Charles C Thomas Publishers, Ltd, Springfield, Illinois, USA.)

References

1. Strichartz GR. Neural physiology and local anesthetic action. In: Cousins MJ, Bridenbaugh PO, eds. Neural blockade in clinical anesthesia and management of pain. 3rd edn. Philadelphia: Lippincott-Raven; 1998: 35–54.
2. Kandel ER, Schwartz JH, Jessel T, eds. Principles of neural science. 2nd edn. New York: Elsevier/North-Holland; 1992.
3. Rang HP, Ritchie JM. On the electrogenic sodium pump in mammalian non-myelinated nerve fibers and its activation by various cations. J Physiol 1968; 196: 183–221.
4. Hille B. Ionic channels of excitable membranes. 2nd edn. Sunderland, MA: Sinauer Associates; 1991.
5. Hodgkin AL, Huxley AF. A quantitative description of membrane current and its application to conduction and excitation in nerve. J Physiol 1952; 117: 500–544.
6. Stühmer W, Conti F, Harukazu S, et al. Structural parts involved in activation and inactivation of the sodium channel. Nature 1989; 339: 565–644.
7. Stoelting RK. Pharmacology and physiology in anesthetic practice. 2nd edn. Philadelphia: JB Lippincott; 1991.
8. Kuhnert PM, Kuhnert BR, Philipson EH, et al. The half-life of 2-chloroprocaine. Anesth Analg 1986; 65: 273–278.
9. O'Brien JE, Abbey V, Hinsvark O, et al. Metabolism and measurement of chloroprocaine, an ester-type local anesthetic. J Pharm Sci 1979; 68: 75–78.
10. DuSouich P, Erill S. Altered metabolism of procainamide and procaine in patients with pulmonary and cardiac diseases. Clin Pharmacol Ther 1977; 21: 101.
11. Reidenberg MM, James M, Dring LG. The rate of procaine hydrolysis in serum of normal subjects and diseased patients. Clin Pharmacol Ther 1972; 13: 279–284.
12. Foldes FF, Davidson GN, Duncalf D, et al. The intravenous toxicity of local anesthetic agents in man. Clin Pharmacol Ther 1965; 40: 328–335.
13. Fisher MM, Graham R. Adverse responses to local anaesthetics. Anaesth Intensive Care 1984; 12: 325–327.
14. Covino BG, Vassalo HL. Local anesthetics: mechanisms of action and clinical use. New York: Grune and Stratton; 1976: 73.
15. Butterworth JF, Strichartz GR. Molecular mechanisms of local anesthesia: a review. Anesthesiology 1990; 72: 711–734.
16. Cahalan M, Shapiro BI, Almers W. Relationship between inactivation of sodium channels and block by quarternary derivatives of local anesthetics and other compounds. In: Fink BR, ed. Molecular mechanisms of anesthesia (Progress in anesthesiology, Vol. 2). New York: Raven Press; 1980.
17. Courtney KR. Structure–activity relations for frequency-dependent sodium channel block in nerve by local anesthetics. J Pharmacol Exp Ther 1980; 213: 114–119.
18. Hille B. Local anesthetics: hydrophilic and hydrophobic pathways for the drug-receptor reaction. J Gen Physiol 1977; 69: 497–515.
19. Hille B. Local anesthetic action on inactivation of the Na^+ channel in nerve and skeletal muscle: possible mechanisms for antiarrhythmic agents. In: Morad M, ed. Biophysical aspects of cardiac muscle. New York: Academic Press; 1978: 55–74.
20. Frazier DT, Narahashi T, Yamada M. The site of action and active form of local anesthetics. II. Experiments with quaternary compounds. J Pharmacol Exp Ther 1970; 171: 45–51.
21. Strichartz GR. The inhibition of sodium currents in myelinated nerve by quaternary derivatives of lidocaine. J Gen Physiol 1973; 62: 37–57.
22. Chernoff DM, Strichartz GR. Tonic and phasic block of neuronal sodium currents by 5-hydroxyhexano-2′,6′-xylidide, a neutral lidocaine homologue. J Gen Physiol 1989; 93: 1075–1090.
23. Ritchie JM, Ritchie BR. Local anaesthetics: effect of pH on activity. Science 1968; 162: 1394–1395.
24. Narahashi T, Frazier D, Yamada M. The site of action and active form of local anesthetics. I. Theory and pH experiments with tertiary compounds. J Pharmacol Exp Ther 1970; 171: 32–44.
25. Sanchez V, Arthur GR, Strichartz G. Fundamental properties of local anesthetics. I. The dependence of lidocaine's ionization and octanol:buffer partitioning on solvent and temperature. Anesth Analg 1987; 66: 159–165.
26. Strichartz GR, Sanchez V, Arthur GR, et al. Fundamental properties of local anesthetics. II. Measured octanol:buffer partition coefficients and pKa values of clinically used drugs. Anesth Analg 1990; 71: 158–170.
27. Truant AP, Takman B. Differential physical-chemical and neuropharmacologic properties of local anesthetic agents. Anesth Analg 1959; 38: 478–484.
28. Tucker GT. Plasma binding and disposition of local anesthetics. Int Anesthesiol Clin 1975; 13: 33–59.
29. Tucker GT, Moore DC, Bridenbaugh PO, et al. Systemic absorption of mepivacaine in commonly used regional block procedures. Anesthesiology 1972; 37; 277–287.
30. Jorfeldt L, Lewis DH, Lofstrom B, et al. Lung uptake of lidocaine in healthy volunteers. Acta Anaesthesiol Scand 1979; 23: 567–574.
31. Lofstrom B. Tissue distribution of local anesthetics with special reference to the lung. Int Anesthesiol Clin 1978; 16: 53–71.
32. Denson DD, Coyle DE, Thompson G, et al. Alpha$_1$-acid glycoprotein and albumin in human serum bupivacaine binding. Clin Pharmacol Ther 1984; 35: 409–415.
33. Kraus E, Polnaszek CF, Scheeler DA, et al. Interaction between human serum albumin and alpha$_1$-acid glycoprotein in the binding of lidocaine to purified protein fractions and sera. J Pharmacol Exp Ther 1986; 239: 754–759.
34. Mather LE, Long GJ, Thomas J. The binding of bupivacaine to maternal and foetal plasma proteins. J Pharm Pharmacol 1971; 23: 359–365.

35. Mather LE, Thomas J. Bupivacaine binding to plasma protein fractions. J Pharm Pharmacol 1978; 30: 653–654.

36. Routledge PA, Barchowsky A, Bjornsson TD, et al. Lidocaine plasma protein binding. Clin Pharmacol Ther 1980; 27: 347–351.

37. Tucker GT, Boyes RN, Bridenbaugh PO, et al. Binding of anilide-type local anesthetics in human plasma. I. Relationships between binding, physiochemical properties and anesthetic activity. Anesthesiology 1970; 33: 287–303.

38. Tucker GT. Pharmacokinetics of local anaesthetics. Br J Anaesth 1986; 58: 717–731.

39. Calvo R, Carlos R, Erill S. Effects of disease and acetazolamine on procaine hydrolysis by red cell enzymes. Clin Pharmacol Ther 1980; 27: 179–183.

40. Javaid JI, Musa MN, Fischman M, et al. Kinetics of cocaine in humans after intravenous and intranasal administration. Biopharm Drug Dispos 1983; 4: 9–18.

41. Tucker GT, Mather LE. Clinical pharmacokinetics of local anaesthetic agents. Clin Pharmacokinet 1979; 4: 241–278.

42. Gissen AJ, Covino BG, Gregus J. Differential sensitivity of mammalian nerve fibers to local anesthetic drugs. Anesthesiology 1980; 53: 467–474.

43. Heinbecker P, Bishop GH, O'Leary J. Pain and touch fibers in peripheral nerves. Arch Neurol Psychiatr 1933; 20: 771–789.

44. Raymond SA, Gissen AJ. Mechanisms of differential block. In: Strichartz GR, ed. Handbook of experimental pharmacology, Vol. 81. Berlin: Springer-Verlag; 1987.

45. de Jong RH. Physiology and pharmacology of local anesthesia. Springfield, IL: Charles C Thomas, 1970.

46. Kristerson L, Nordenram Å, Nordqvist P. Penetration of radioactive local anaesthetic into peripheral nerve. Arch Int Pharmacodyn 1965; 157: 148–151.

47. Winnie AP, LaVallee DA, Sosa BP, et al. Clinical pharmacokinetics of local anesthetics. Can Anaesth Soc J 1977; 24: 252.

48. Winnie AP, Tay CH, Patel KP, et al. Pharmacokinetics of local anesthetics during plexus blocks. Anesth Analg 1977; 56: 852–861.

CHAPTER 4

General indications and contraindications

PERIPHERAL NERVE BLOCK: INDICATIONS

Surgery

"A thorough knowledge of descriptive and topographic anatomy, especially with regard to nerve distribution, is beyond discussion. It is a condition which anyone desirous of attempting the study of regional anesthesia should fulfil. The anatomy of the human body must, besides, be approached from an angle hitherto unknown to the medical student and with which the average surgeon is not at all familiar."[1]

Gaston Labat wrote these words at a time when deep ether anesthesia was required to provide adequate muscle relaxation, especially for abdominal surgery. The problems associated with deep ether anesthesia included nausea, vomiting, and atelectasis and subsequent pneumonia. Therefore the benefits of regional anesthesia were readily apparent. The practice of regional anesthesia still holds attraction, possibly because of its positive effects on secondary outcomes such as postoperative nausea and vomiting, postoperative confusion, and rapid return to 'street fitness'. Evidence of a positive influence on the 'hard' postoperative outcomes of morbidity and mortality is more difficult to come by, although a number of studies have shown benefit in specific circumstances.[2–4] Practicing regional anesthesia is also an opportunity for anesthesiologists to employ their individual skills, and so can be an important source of professional satisfaction. Practitioners are responsible for acquainting themselves with the anatomy

to which Labat refers and to which a large part of this textbook and DVD-ROM is directed. This knowledge lies at the core of successful regional anesthetic practice and the avoidance of many of its complications.

The dermatomes and myotomes of the body and limbs are shown in Figs 4.1–4.9. The selection of a regional anesthetic technique appropriate to a particular surgical intervention becomes more straightforward when one can answer the following questions:

- What dermatomes, myotomes, and osteotomes are involved?
- Will a tourniquet be used to provide a bloodless field?
- How much pain can be expected in the postoperative period?
- Is the surgery to be performed on an ambulatory basis?
- Is there a specific contraindication to the proposed technique?
- Are both surgeon and patient in agreement with the proposed technique?

Management of acute pain

Pain arises from the direct activation of primary afferent neurons. It is often associated with tissue damage and an inflammatory response, especially in the clinical setting. The inflammatory response has both cellular and neurogenic components. Activation of lymphocytes, macrophages, and mast cells, and the release of neuropeptides such as substance P and neurokinin A result in the further release of inflammatory

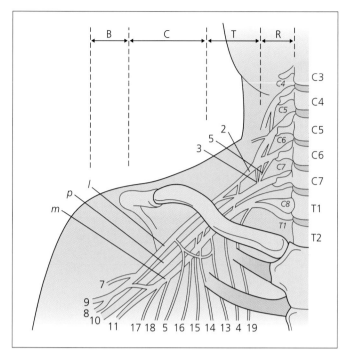

Figure 4.1 Brachial plexus.
R, roots (ventral rami of spinal nerves); T, trunks (superior, middle, and inferior); C, cords (lateral, posterior, and medial); B, terminal branches; P, pectoralis minor muscle.
1, Dorsal scapular nerve; 2, suprascapular nerve; 3, nerve to subclavius muscle; 4, superior pectoral nerve; 5, lateral pectoral nerve; 6, axillary artery; 7, musculocutaneous nerve; 8, median nerve; 9, axillary nerve; 10, radial nerve; 11, ulnar nerve; 12, axillary vein; 13, medial pectoral nerve; 14, superior subscapular nerve; 15, thoracodorsal (middle subscapular) nerve; 16, inferior subscapular nerve; 17, medial cutaneous nerve of the forearm; 18, medial cutaneous nerve of the arm; 19, long thoracic nerve.

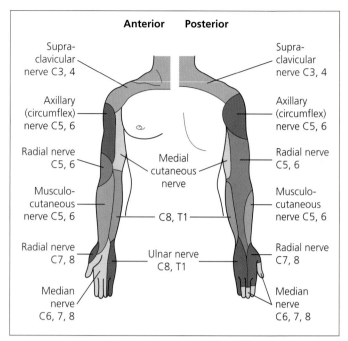

Figure 4.2 Cutaneous innervation of the upper limb.

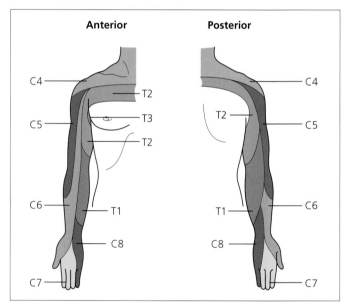

Figure 4.3 Dermatomes of the upper limb.

mediators such as histamine, bradykinin, and the products of arachidonic acid metabolism.[6–9] These chemicals can sensitize high-threshold nociceptors to produce the phenomenon of *peripheral sensitization*. The resultant area of primary hyperalgesia is characterized by an increased responsiveness to thermal and low-threshold mechanical stimuli at the site of injury.

In addition to the area of primary hyperalgesia, a zone of secondary hyperalgesia develops in the uninjured tissues surrounding the site of injury. No changes occur in the threshold to stimuli of the nerves in this area; rather, it is changes occurring in the dorsal horn of the spinal cord that are thought responsible for this *central sensitization*.[10] Changes that occur in the dorsal horn in association with central sensitization include an expansion in receptive field size, increased response to stimuli, and a reduction in threshold. These changes are important in both acute pain and the development of chronic pain.[11,12]

Non-steroidal anti-inflammatory drugs (NSAIDs) exert their action by blocking the cyclo-oxygenase (COX) enzyme pathway. With traditional agents, this has involved the inhibition of both the COX_1 and COX_2 isoforms. Reductions in pain scores and opioid requirements have been reported with their use. The COX_2 isoform is predominantly induced by the inflammatory process, and the recent development and introduction into clinical practice of specific COX_2 inhibitors,

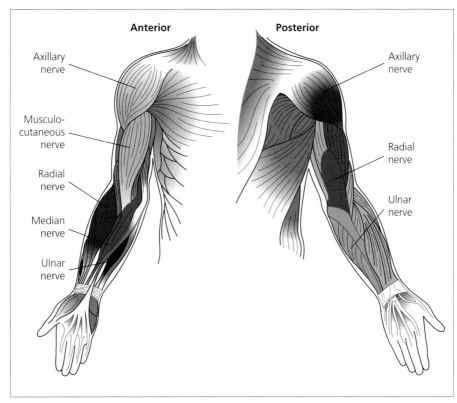

Figure 4.4 Myotomes of the upper limb.

holds promise for a reduction in side effects of these drugs.[13] Evidence also exists to support a central mechanism of action of NSAIDs in the modification of pain mechanisms.[14]

The role of opioid drugs in the modification of central pain mechanisms has been long recognized. They act presynaptically to inhibit the release of neurotransmitters from the nociceptive primary afferent neuron. Peripheral nerves are known to manufacture opioid receptors in the cell body and transport them to both the periphery and the dorsal horn. Following tissue injury, the peripheral receptors become active.[15,16] Initial interest in exploiting these features has waned somewhat as equivocal results following the intra-articular administration of morphine to treat arthroscopic procedure-related pain have been published.[17]

Damage to peripheral nerves results in pathophysiologic changes in the nerves themselves.[18] Such damage manifests as spontaneous firing, increased sensitivity to non-noxious stimuli, demyelination, and the sprouting of nerve fibers. These changes form the basis for the development of peripheral chronic pain states. Low concentrations of local anesthetic can reduce ectopic activity in damaged nerves, a feature utilized during their systemic administration for the treatment of neuropathic pain.[19] Local anesthetic field block combined with wound infiltration has been shown to significantly reduce pain scores and opioid requirements for up

to a week following hernia repair.[20] Wound infiltration is an integral part of this technique; however, definitive evidence showing prevention in the development of the above changes remains lacking.

The concept and effectiveness of pre-emptive analgesia remain controversial.[21] At its heart, however, is the hypothesis that the prevention of noxious inputs occurring during and after surgery will prevent the development of central sensitization. While it has been demonstrated that early postoperative pain is a predictor of long-term pain, it is not known what degree of noxious input is required, or for how long it must be present to produce long-term changes in the nervous system.[22] The logic of combining NSAIDs, opioids, and a regional anesthetic technique (with or without perineural catheter) appears self-evident, yet definitive evidence of benefit in the clinical setting is lacking and the standardization of study methods is required to allow firm conclusions to be drawn.[23–25]

Chronic pain

The indications for somatic peripheral nerve block in the management of chronic pain are limited, and the results require careful interpretation. A common indication has been to determine the likelihood of success following surgical decompression or neurolysis of a peripheral nerve. Small

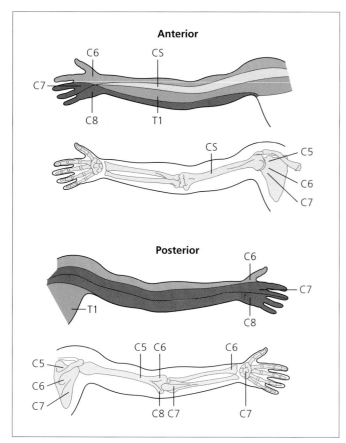

Figure 4.5 Osseous innervation of the upper limb.

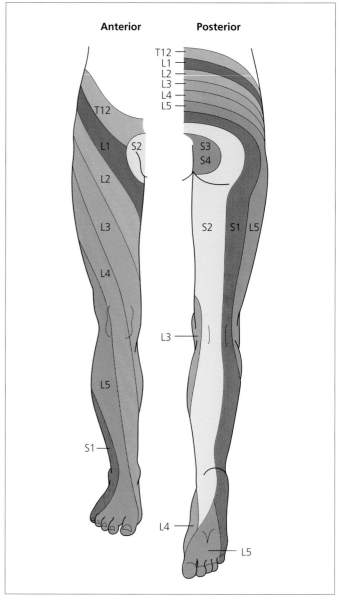

Figure 4.6 Dermatomes of the lower limb.

volumes of local anesthetic need to be used in this setting to prevent spread to other nerves, and long-acting agents allow one to differentiate the results from the placebo effect, which in itself tends to be short-lived.[26]

CONTINUOUS NERVE BLOCK

Continuous catheter techniques are gaining widespread use in a number of clinical settings. These include acute pain relief in the inpatient and ambulatory settings, early postoperative rehabilitation, continuous sympathectomy following re-implantation procedures, and the diagnosis and treatment of chronic pain syndromes.[27–31] Indeed, there have been published reports of improved surgical outcomes with these techniques, in addition to improved secondary outcomes.[32]

The concerns regarding continuous techniques have related to infection, catheter migration, high plasma levels of local anesthetic, local myelotoxicity, and neurologic complications. Infection has been reported, yet despite a colonization rate of up to 27%, overt problems appear to be rare.[33] Catheter migra-

tion can be detected early with regular and routine examination of catheter site and assessment of the nerve block.

Plasma levels of local anesthetic may rise progressively during an infusion. Although the perioperative rise in α_1-acid glycoprotein (GP) has been shown to ameliorate the effect, a seizure rate of 1.2 per 1000 procedures has been reported.[34,35] Postoperative protocols, education of carers, and patient cooperation are necessary to detect the early signs of local anesthetic toxicity and ensure the optimal use of this technology.

The incidence of neurologic complications is less than 1% with the use of perineural catheters. This is similar to the

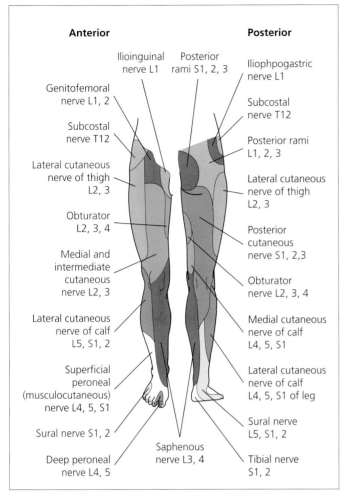

Figure 4.7 Cutaneous innervation of the lower limb.

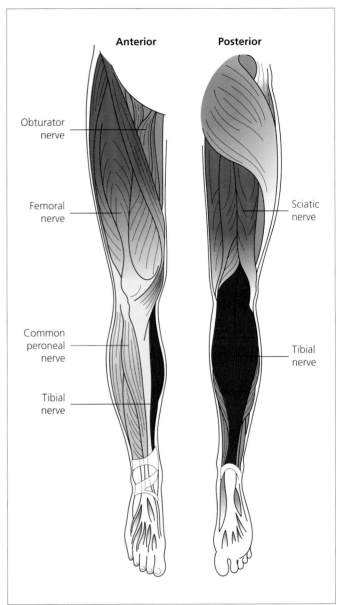

Figure 4.8 Muscular innervation of the lower limb.

rates recorded following multiple single-dose techniques.[36] Whether the incidence of complications can be reduced further using ultrasound to guide catheter placement remains to be seen. It should be noted that catheter techniques are often used in major joint surgery such as distraction inter-position arthroplasty, which carries an inherent high risk of nerve injury.[37]

PERIPHERAL NERVE BLOCK: CONTRAINDICATIONS

Anticoagulant medication

Hematoma formation following peripheral nerve block is considered to be uncommon and usually of little importance. However, it can produce significant patient discomfort, persistent paresthesias, and occasionally be severe and extensive. The administration of anticoagulant medication is a risk factor

for the development of prolonged bleeding following venous or arterial puncture. Precautions to be observed for the perioperative use of anticoagulants have been outlined by the American Society of Regional Anesthesia and Pain Medicine (see Guidelines, p. 24) as well as equivalent organizations outside the USA.[38] These guidelines have been informed by the contrasting US and European experiences in neuraxial block, specifically in relation to the occurrence of spinal and epidural hematoma. Until and unless further studies suggest otherwise, it appears prudent to observe the same recommendations when performing peripheral nerve block, particularly if the nerves are deep or lie in proximity to non-compressible vessels.

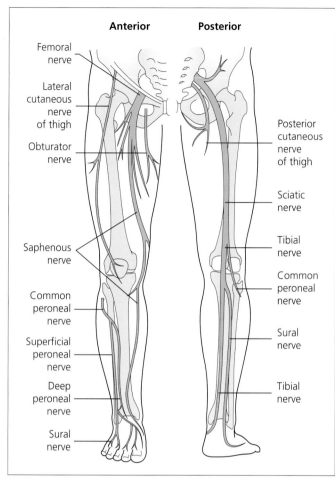

Figure 4.9 The main nerves of the lower limb.

Heparin

Intravenous heparin has a half-life of $1\frac{1}{2}$–2 h and is cleared within 4–6 h of administration. It stimulates the formation of antithrombin III, which forms a complex with activated thrombin, thus neutralizing thrombin activity and preventing the conversion of fibrinogen to fibrin. Its effects can be reversed with protamine; 1 mg per 100 U of heparin.

Protamine forms an inactive complex with heparin. The activity of heparin can be measured with the activated partial thromboplastin time (APTT) and the activated clotting time, both being sensitive tests of heparin function. There is a wide variation in dose responses between individuals; this variation is further affected by diet, liver function, renal function, and cardiac status.[40] Laboratory testing should be performed on patients who have received heparin prior to nerve block.

Subcutaneous heparin, 5000 U 12 hourly, displays maximal activity at 50 min and is effective for 4–6 h. The APTT very often remains unchanged. Low molecular weight heparin (LMWH), however, has a higher bioavailability, longer half-life, and smaller effect on platelet function.

Non-inflammatory anti-inflammatory drugs

The NSAIDs inhibit thromboxane synthesis as well as the release of adenosine diphosphate by platelets and their subsequent aggregation. This effect is permanent in the case of aspirin and lasts the lifetime of the platelet (approximately 10 days).

Coumarin derivatives

The coumarin derivatives, principally warfarin, inhibit synthesis of vitamin K-dependent clotting factors (II, VII, IX, and X). The international normalized ratio (INR) may not reflect levels of factors II and X for some time following the discontinuation of warfarin. Vitamin K reverses warfarin's effects, although doses up to 50 mg may be required for complete reversal. For elective surgery, discontinuation of warfarin 3–4 days prior to surgery is usually sufficient. For acute reversal, fresh frozen plasma and factor concentrates will achieve the same end.

New anticoagulants

The hirudin derivatives inhibit free and clot-bound thrombin, and fondaparinux inhibits factor Xa. These newer drugs are becoming more widely used, but the risk of neuraxial hematoma is unknown.

Guidelines – Regional anesthesia in the anticoagulated patient: defining the risks

Anesthetic management of the patient receiving thrombolytic therapy

Patients receiving fibrinolytic or thrombolytic medications are at risk of serious hemorrhagic events, particularly those who have undergone an invasive procedure. Consensus statements are based on the profound effect on hemostasis, the use of concomitant heparin and/or antiplatelet agents (that further increase the risk of bleeding), and the potential for spontaneous neuraxial bleeding with these medications.

Advances in fibrinolytic and thrombolytic therapy have been associated with an increased use of these drugs, which will require further increases in vigilance. Ideally, the patient should be queried prior to the thrombolytic therapy for a recent history of lumbar puncture, spinal or epidural anesthesia, or epidural steroid injection to allow appropriate monitoring. Guidelines detailing original contraindications for thrombolytic drugs suggest avoidance of these drugs for 10 days following puncture of non-compressible vessels.

Preoperative evaluation should determine whether fibrinolytic or thrombolytic drugs have been used preoperatively, or have the likelihood of being used intraoperatively or postoperatively. Patients receiving fibrinolytic and thrombolytic drugs should be cautioned against receiving spinal or epidural anesthetics except in highly unusual circumstances. Data are not available to clearly outline the length of time neuraxial puncture should be avoided after discontinuation of these drugs.

In those patients who have received neuraxial blocks at or near the time of fibrinolytic and thrombolytic therapy, neurologic monitoring should be continued for an appropriate interval. It may be that the interval of monitoring should not be more than 2 h between neurologic checks. Furthermore, if neuraxial blocks have been combined with fibrinolytic and thrombolytic therapy and ongoing epidural catheter infusion, the infusion should be limited to drugs minimizing sensory and motor block to facilitate assessment of neurologic function.

There is no definitive recommendation for removal of neuraxial catheters in patients who unexpectedly receive fibrinolytic and thrombolytic therapy during a neuraxial catheter infusion. The measurement of fibrinogen level (one of the last clotting factors to recover) may be helpful in making a decision about catheter removal or maintenance.

Anesthetic management of the patient receiving unfractionated heparin

Anesthetic management of the heparinized patient was established over two decades ago. Initial recommendations have been supported by in-depth reviews of case series, case reports of spinal hematoma, and the American Society of Anesthesiologists Closed Claims Project.

During subcutaneous (minidose) prophylaxis there is no contraindication to the use of neuraxial techniques. The risk of neuraxial bleeding may be reduced by delay of the heparin injection until after the block, and may be increased in debilitated patients after prolonged therapy. Since heparin-induced thrombocytopenia may occur during heparin administration, patients receiving heparin for greater than 4 days should have a platelet count assessed prior to neuraxial block and catheter removal.

Combining neuraxial techniques with intraoperative anticoagulation with heparin during vascular surgery seems acceptable with the following cautions:

- Avoid the technique in patients with other coagulopathies.
- Heparin administration should be delayed for 1 h after needle placement.
- Indwelling neuraxial catheters should be removed 2–4 h after the last heparin dose and the patient's coagulation status is evaluated; reheparinization should occur 1 h after catheter removal.
- Monitor the patient postoperatively to provide early detection of motor blockade and consider use of minimal concentration of local anesthetics to enhance the early detection of a spinal hematoma.
- Although the occurrence of a bloody or difficult neuraxial needle placement may increase risk, there are no data to support mandatory cancellation of a case. Direct communication with the surgeon and a specific risk–benefit decision about proceeding in each case is warranted.

Currently, insufficient data and experience are available to determine if the risk of neuraxial hematoma is increased when combining neuraxial techniques with the full anticoagulation of cardiac surgery. Postoperative monitoring of neurologic function and selection of neuraxial solutions that minimize sensory and motor block is recommended to facilitate detection of new or progressive neurodeficits.

The concurrent use of medications that affect other components of the clotting mechanisms may increase the risk of bleeding complications for patients receiving standard heparin. These medications include antiplatelet medications, LMWH, and oral anticoagulants.

Anesthetic management of the patient receiving low molecular weight heparin

Anesthesiologists in North America can draw on the extensive European experience to develop practice guidelines for the management of patients undergoing spinal and epidural blocks while receiving perioperative LMWH. All consensus statements contained herein respect the labeled dosing regimens of LMWH as established by the US Food and Drugs Administration (FDA). Although it is impossible to devise recommendations that will completely eliminate the risk of spinal hematoma, previous consensus recommendations have appeared to improve outcome. Concern remains for higher-dose applications, where sustained therapeutic levels of anticoagulation are present.

Monitoring of the anti-Xa level is not recommended. The anti-Xa level is not predictive of the risk of bleeding and is, therefore, not helpful in the management of patients undergoing neuraxial blocks.

Antiplatelet or oral anticoagulant medications administered in combination with LMWH may increase the risk of spinal hematoma. Concomitant administration of medications affecting hemostasis, such as antiplatelet drugs, standard heparin, or dextran, represents an additional risk of hemorrhagic complications perioperatively, including spinal hematoma. Education of the entire patient-care team is necessary to avoid potentiation of the anticoagulant effects.

The presence of blood during needle and catheter placement does not necessitate postponement of surgery. However, initiation of LMWH therapy in this setting should be delayed for 24 h postoperatively. Traumatic needle or catheter placement may signify an increased risk of spinal hematoma, and it is recommended that this consideration be discussed with the surgeon.

Preoperative LMWH
- Patients on preoperative LMWH thromboprophylaxis can be assumed to have altered coagulation. In these patients needle placement should occur at least 10–12 h after the LMWH dose.
- Patients receiving higher (treatment) doses of LMWH, such as enoxaparin 1 mg/kg every 12 h, enoxaparin 1.5 mg/kg daily, dalteparin 120 U/kg every 12 h, dalteparin 200 U/kg daily, or tinzaparin 175 U/kg daily will require delays of at least 24 h to assure normal hemostasis at the time of needle insertion.
- Neuraxial techniques should be avoided in patients administered a dose of LMWH 2 h preoperatively (general surgery patients), because needle placement would occur during peak anticoagulant activity.

Postoperative LMWH
Patients with postoperative initiation of LMWH thromboprophylaxis may safely undergo single-injection and continuous catheter techniques. Management is based on total daily dose, timing of the first postoperative dose, and dosing schedule.

Twice-daily dosing
This dosage regimen may be associated with an increased risk of spinal hematoma. The first dose of LMWH should be administered no earlier than 24 h postoperatively, regardless of anesthetic technique, and only in the presence of adequate (surgical) hemostasis. Indwelling catheters should be removed prior to initiation of LMWH thromboprophylaxis. If a continuous technique is selected, the epidural catheter may be left indwelling overnight and removed the following day, with the first dose of LMWH administered 2 h after catheter removal.

Single daily dosing
This dosing regimen approximates the European application. The first postoperative LMWH dose should be administered 6–8 h postoperatively. The second postoperative dose should occur no sooner than 24 h after the first dose. Indwelling neuraxial catheters may be safely maintained. However, the catheter should be removed a minimum of 10–12 h after the last dose of LMWH. Subsequent LMWH dosing should occur a minimum of 2 h after catheter removal.

Regional anesthetic management of the patient on oral anticoagulants

The management of patients receiving warfarin perioperatively remains controversial. Consensus statements are based on warfarin pharmacology, the clinical relevance of vitamin K coagulation factor levels and deficiencies, and the case reports of spinal hematoma among these patients.

Caution should be used when performing neuraxial techniques in patients recently discontinued from chronic warfarin therapy. The anticoagulant therapy must be stopped (ideally 4–5 days prior to the planned procedure), and the prothrombin time (PT)/INR measured prior to initiation of neuraxial block. Early after discontinuation of

warfarin therapy. The anticoagulant therapy must be stopped (ideally 4–5 days prior to the planned procedure), and the prothrombin time (PT)/INR measured prior to initiation of neuraxial block. Early after discontinuation of warfarin therapy, the PT/INR reflect predominantly factor VII levels, and despite acceptable factor VII levels, factors II and X levels may not be adequate for normal hemostasis. Adequate levels of II, VII, IX, and X may not be present until the PT/INT is within normal limits.

The concurrent use of medications that affect other components of the clotting mechanisms may increase the risk of bleeding complications for patients receiving oral anticoagulants, and do so without influencing the PT/INR. These medications include aspirin and other NSAIDs, ticlopidine and clopidogrel, unfractionated heparin, and LMWH.

For patients receiving an initial dose of warfarin prior to surgery, the PT/INR should be checked prior to neuraxial block if the first dose was given more than 24 h earlier, or a second dose of oral anticoagulant has been administered.

Patients receiving low-dose warfarin therapy during epidural analgesia should have their PT/INR monitored on a daily basis, and checked before catheter removal, if initial doses of warfarin are administered more than 36 h preoperatively. Initial studies evaluating the safety of epidural analgesia in association with oral anticoagulation utilized mean daily doses of approximately 5 mg of warfarin. Higher dose warfarin may require more intensive monitoring of the coagulation status.

As thromboprophylaxis with warfarin is initiated, neuraxial catheters should be removed when the INR is < 1.5. This value was derived from studies correlating hemostasis with clotting factor activity levels greater than 40%.

Neurologic testing of sensory and motor function should be performed routinely during epidural analgesia for patients on warfarin therapy. The type of analgesic solution should be tailored to minimize the degree of sensory and motor blockade. These checks should be continued after catheter removal for at least 24 h, and longer if the INR was greater than 1.5 at the time of catheter removal.

An INR > 3 should prompt the physician to withhold or reduce the warfarin dose in patients with indwelling neuraxial catheters. We can make no definitive recommendation for removal of neuraxial catheters in patients with therapeutic levels of anticoagulation during neuraxial catheter infusion.

Reduced doses of warfarin should be given to patients who are likely to have an enhanced response to the drug.

Anesthetic management of the patient receiving antiplatelet medications

Antiplatelet medications, including NSAIDs, thienopyridine derivatives (ticlopidine and clopidogrel), and platelet GP IIb/IIIa antagonists (abciximab, eptifibatide, and tirofiban) exert diverse effects on platelet function. The pharmacologic differences make it impossible to extrapolate between the groups of drugs regarding the practice of neuraxial techniques.

There is no wholly accepted test, including the bleeding time, which will guide antiplatelet therapy. Careful preoperative assessment of the patient to identify alterations of health that might contribute to bleeding is crucial. These conditions include a history of easy bruisability or excessive bleeding, female gender, and increased age.

The NSAIDs appear to represent no added significant risk for the development of spinal hematoma in patients having epidural or spinal anesthesia. The use of NSAIDs alone does not create a level of risk that will interfere with the performance of neuraxial blocks.

At this time, there do not seem to be specific concerns as to the timing of single-shot or catheter techniques in relationship to the dosing of NSAIDs, postoperative monitoring, or the timing of neuraxial catheter removal.

The actual risk of spinal hematoma with ticlopidine and clopidogrel and the GP IIb/IIIa antagonists is unknown. Consensus management is based on labeling precautions and the surgical, interventional cardiology and radiology experience.

- Based on labeling and surgical reviews, the suggested time interval between discontinuation of thienopyridine therapy and neuraxial blockade is 14 days for ticlopidine and 7 days for clopidogrel.
- Platelet GP IIb/IIIa inhibitors exert a profound effect on platelet aggregation. Following administration, the time to normal platelet aggregation is 24–48 h for abciximab and 4–8 h for eptifibatide and tirofiban. Neuraxial techniques should be avoided until platelet function has recovered. GP IIb/IIIa antagonists are contraindicated within 4 weeks of surgery. Should one be administered in the postoperative period (following a neuraxial technique), the patient should be carefully monitored neurologically.

The concurrent use of other medications affecting clotting mechanisms, such as oral anticoagulants, unfractionated heparin, and LMWH, may increase the risk of bleeding complications. Cyclooxygenase-2 inhibitors have minimal effect on platelet function and should be considered in patients who require anti-inflammatory therapy in the presence of anticoagulation.

Anesthetic management of the patient receiving herbal therapy

Herbal drugs, by themselves, appear to represent no added significant risk for the development of spinal hematoma in patients having epidural or spinal anesthesia. This is an important observation because it is likely that a significant number of our surgical patients utilize alternative medications preoperatively and perhaps during their postoperative course.

The use of herbal medications alone does not create a level of risk that will interfere with the performance of neuraxial blocks. Mandatory discontinuation of these medications, or cancellation of surgery in patients in whom these medications have been continued, is not supported by available data.

Data on the combination of herbal therapy with other forms of anticoagulation are lacking. However, the concurrent use of other medications affecting clotting mechanisms, such as oral anticoagulants or heparin, may increase the risk of bleeding complications in these patients.

There is no wholly accepted test to assess adequacy of hemostasis in the patient reporting preoperative herbal medications.

At this time, there do not seem to be specific concerns as to the timing of neuraxial block in relationship to the dosing of herbal therapy, postoperative monitoring, or the timing of neuraxial catheter removal.

New Anticoagulants

New antithrombotic drugs, which target various steps in the hemostatic system, such as inhibiting platelet aggregation, blocking coagulation factors, or enhancing fibrinolysis, are continually under development. The most extensively studied are antagonists of specific platelet receptors and direct thrombin inhibitors. Many of these antithrombotic agents have prolonged half-lives and are difficult to reverse without administration of blood components. It is likely that orally bioavailable 'heparins' will be introduced in the near future. The administration of these medications in combination with neuraxial anesthesia must be carefully considered.

Thrombin Inhibitors

Recombinant hirudin derivatives, including desirudin (Revasc, Aventis Pharmaceuticals, Paris, France), lepirudin (Refludan, Aventis Pharmaceuticals), and bivalirudin (Angiomax, The Medicine Co., Cambridge, MA) inhibit both free and clot-bound thrombin. Argatroban (Acova), an L-arginine derivative, has a similar mechanism of action. These medications are indicated for the treatment and prevention of thrombosis in patients with heparin-induced thrombocytopenia and as an adjunct to angioplasty procedures. Desirudin has also been evaluated for prevention of DVT/PE following hip replacement. The anticoagulant effect of thrombin inhibitors is monitored by the aPTT, and is present for 1 to 3 hours after IV administration. Hemorrhagic complications, particularly when combined with thrombolytic or antiplatelet agents, may be life threatening. There is no 'antidote'; the antithrombin effect cannot be reversed pharmacologically. Although there are no case reports of spinal hematoma related to neuraxial anesthesia among patients who have received a thrombin inhibitor, spontaneous intracranial bleeding has been reported. Due to the lack of information available, no statement regarding risk assessment and patient management can be made. Identification of cardiology and surgical risk factors associated with bleeding following invasive procedures may be helpful.

Fondaparinux

Fondaparinux, an injectable synthetic pentasaccharide, was approved in December 2001. The FDA released fondaparinux (Arixtra, Sanofi-Synthelabo, West Orange, NJ) with a black box warning similar to that of the LMWHs and heparinoids. Fondaparinux produces its antithrombotic effect through factor Xa inhibition. The plasma half-life of fondaparinux is 21 hours, allowing for single daily dosing, with the first dose administered 6 hours postoperatively. Investigators reported a spinal hematoma among the initial dose-ranging study (at a dose that was subsequently determined to be twice required for thromboprophylaxis). No additional spinal hematomas were reported in the combined series of 3,600 patients who underwent spinal or epidural anesthesia in combination with fondaparinux thromboprophylaxis. However, the conditions for performance of neuraxial block were strictly controlled. Patients were included in subsequent clinical trials only if needle placement was atraumatic and accomplished on the first attempt. In addition, indwelling epidural catheters were removed 2 hours prior to fondaparinux administration. These practice guidelines may not be feasible in clinical practice. For example, in a prospective series, less than 40% of neuraxial blocks were successful with one pass.

Guidelines – Regional anesthesia in the anticoagulated patient: defining the risks

Anesthetic Management of the Patient Receiving Fondaparinux

The actual risk of spinal hematoma with fondaparinux is unknown. Consensus statements are based on the sustained and irreversible antithrombotic effect, early postoperative dosing, and the spinal hematoma reported during initial clinical trials. Close monitoring of the surgical literature for risk factors associated with surgical bleeding may be helpful in risk assessment and patient management. Until further clinical experience is available, performance of neuraxial techniques should occur under conditions utilized in clinical trials (single needle pass, atraumatic needle placement, avoidance of indwelling neuraxial catheters). If this is not feasible, an alternate method of prophylaxis should be considered.

(From: Horlocker TT, Wedel DJ, Benzon H, et al. Regional anesthesia in the anticoagulated patient: defining the risks (the second ASRA Consensus Conference on Neuraxial Anesthesia and Anticoagulation). Reg Anesth Pain Med. 2003; 28: 172-97, with permission from the American Society of Regional Anesthesia and Pain Medicine.)

Respiratory disease

The phrenic nerve (C3, 4, 5) is a branch of the cervical plexus, its three roots usually joining at the lateral border of scalenus anterior muscle. The nerve passes across the anterior aspect of the muscle and descends to enter the thorax, having passed between subclavian artery and vein. The incidence of ipsilateral phrenic nerve paresis following supraclavicular block ranges from 36%, regardless of technique used, to 100% with the interscalene approach.[41,42] With ultrasonographic assessment, this 100% incidence remains despite a reduction in the mass of local anesthetic used. A 25% reduction in forced vital capacity (FVC) and forced expiratory volume in 1 s (FEV_1), as well as a reduction in peak expiratory flow rate (PEFR), can be expected following interscalene block. This persists for the duration of action of the anesthetic agent.[43,44] The patient with normal pulmonary function can tolerate this embarrassment easily. However, those with poor respiratory reserve are at risk of developing acute respiratory failure. The wisdom of performing these blocks in such patients must be questioned, and bilateral blocks are absolutely contra-indicated. An $FEV_1 < 1$ L, FVC < 15–20 mL/kg, FEV/FVC $< 35\%$, PEFR < 100 L/min, and $pCO_2 > 50$ mmHg are predictors of serious respiratory compromise following supraclavicular block.[45] Further absolute contraindications to interscalene brachial plexus block include a history of pre-existing contralateral hemidiaphragmatic paralysis or contralateral pneumonectomy.

Any procedure in which a needle is directed toward the lung carries a risk of pneumothorax. The incidence of pneumothorax with supraclavicular blocks has variously been reported as being 6–25%.[46,47] A sudden cough or inspiratory effort should alert the operator to the possibility of pneumothorax, because the symptoms and signs may not develop for hours or until the pneumothorax reaches 20% of lung volume. Radiographic evidence may take 24 h to develop.

The performance of intercostal or paravertebral nerve block for analgesia is preferable to no analgesia or high-dose narcotics, especially in the elderly. Dilute solutions sufficient to provide analgesia without significant motor blockade should be advocated, because case reports of respiratory failure secondary to intercostal motor block and without pneumothorax following intercostal block have appeared.[48,49]

Neuromuscular disease

Pre-existing or unstable neuromuscular disease is often considered to be a contraindication to regional anesthesia. These patients, however, are very often at increased risk of respiratory failure, autonomic dysfunction, and myocardial dysfunction in the perioperative period. They should have a detailed neurologic assessment documented, as well as an appropriate assessment of other body systems that may be affected by the disease process. Changes in the perioperative period are often seen in these patients as a consequence of fatigue, stress, and infection. A careful risk–benefit analysis may, nevertheless, allow the anesthesiologist to affect positively the postoperative outcome of these patients.

Multiple sclerosis

Multiple sclerosis is a demyelinating disease of the brain and spinal cord characterized by a series of remissions and exacerbations occurring over many years. Multiple sclerosis does not affect the peripheral nervous system. Epidural and, more especially, spinal anesthesia have been implicated in exacerbations of multiple sclerosis.[50] Theories to explain this suggest that demyelinated nerves may be more susceptible to the neurotoxic effects of local anesthetic agents.[51] While peripheral nerve block is performed at a 'safe' distance from the disease process of multiple sclerosis, there always exists the potential for exacerbations secondary to stress or infection in the perioperative period. Patients should be informed of this and their neurologic status documented before and after any intervention.

Amyotrophic lateral sclerosis

Amyotrophic lateral sclerosis is a degenerative disease of upper and lower motor neurons and the motor nuclei of the brainstem. Its cause is unknown. Amyotrophic lateral sclerosis is associated with bulbar muscle weakness, the risk of aspiration, autonomic system dysfunction, and poor ventilatory reserve. Little information exists on the safety of performing peripheral nerve blocks in patients with amyotrophic lateral sclerosis. Epidural block has been successfully employed, suggesting that it may be safe to use local anesthetic agents in this group.[52]

Myasthenia gravis

Myasthenia gravis is an autoimmune disease affecting the neuromuscular junction. Up to 90% of myasthenia patients have anti-acetylcholine receptor antibodies, and the disease is characterized by skeletal muscle weakness exacerbated by activity. Patients with myasthenia are extremely sensitive to non-depolarizing neuromuscular-blocking drugs. In addition, the relaxant effects of volatile anesthetic agents are markedly pronounced in these patients, and reduced plasma cholinesterase activity may prolong the elimination half-life of ester local anesthetics.

The following factors identify patients at high risk of respiratory compromise and the need for postoperative ventilation:[53]

- the presence of disease for 6 years or more;
- a vital capacity of less than 2.9 L;
- coexisting chronic obstructive airway disease; and
- a pyridostigmine requirement of more than 750 mg/day.

Peripheral nerve block is an obvious choice of anesthetic technique in these patients, unless it carries the risk of interfering with respiratory or bulbar function.

Guillain–Barré syndrome

Guillain–Barré syndrome is an acute demyelinating disease of the peripheral nervous system. An autoimmune mechanism following a recent viral illness is thought to be responsible. It is characterized by the cephalad progression of flaccid paralysis, respiratory weakness, and bulbar and autonomic dysfunction; 20% of patients have residual neurologic deficits. Epidural anesthesia has been employed successfully in this population, although the hemodynamic changes that may occur and an exaggerated response to indirect vasopressors may render this a high-risk intervention.[54]

Diabetes mellitus

Diabetes is a disease that produces multiorgan dysfunction. In many respects it may be preferable to proceed with a regional anesthesia technique in these patients. The risk of perioperative myocardial ischemia, hypoglycemia, autonomic dysfunction, and possible difficult intubation would make this so. Unfortunately, the peripheral neuropathy common to diabetes may involve the area to be blocked. Careful mapping of any neurologic deficit is therefore necessary. Motor responses may be difficult to elicit at normal nerve stimulator settings, and sensation may not be fully intact, heightening the

risk of nerve injury. In addition, coma, secondary to a central conduction block of the normal physiologic response to hypoglycemia, has been reported.[55] This further highlights the dangers faced by patients with diabetes.

Box 4.1 Contraindications to peripheral nerve block	
Absolute	**Relative**
Patient refusal	Respiratory compromise
Local infection	as outlined
Full anticoagulation	Neuromuscular disease
Allergy to local anesthetic	as outlined
	Diabetes

SUMMARY

The contraindications to peripheral nerve block are broadly summarized in Box 4.1. The reader is advised to consult the text relating to specific blocks for further detail of individual contraindications.

References

1. Labat G. Regional anesthesia: techniques and clinical applications. Philadelphia: WB Saunders; 1922: 2.
2. Sorensen RM, Pace NL. Anesthetic techniques during surgical repair of femoral neck fractures: a meta-analysis. Anesthesiology 1992; 77: 1095–1104.
3. Urwin SC, Parker MJ, Griffiths R. General versus regional anesthesia for hip fracture surgery: a meta-analysis of randomized trials. Br J Anaesth 2000; 84: 450–455.
4. Sharrock NE, Cazan MG, Hargett MJL, et al. Changes in mortality after total hip and knee arthroplasty over a ten year period. Anesth Analg 1995; 80: 242–248.
5. Gaertner E, Navez M-L, Aknin P, et al. Anesthésie régionale: anesthésie tronculaire et plexique de l'adulte. Paris: Arnette Groupe Liaisons; 2001: 58–63.
6. Levine JD, Fields HL, Basbaum AI. Peptides and the primary afferent nociceptor. J Neurosci 1993; 13: 2273–2286.
7. Dray A, Urban L, Dickenson A. Pharmacology of chronic pain. Trends Pharmacol Sci 1994;15: 190–197.
8. Forster RW, Ramage AG. The action of some chemical irritants on somatosensory receptors of the cat. Neuropharmacology 1981; 20: 191–198.
9. Perl ER. Sensitization of nociceptors and its relation to sensation. In: Bonica JJ, AlbeFessard D, eds. Advances in pain research and therapy. New York: Raven Press; 1976: 17–28.
10. Bennett GJ, Kajander KC, Sahara Y, et al. Neurochemical and anatomical changes in the dorsal horn of rats with an experimental painful peripheral neuropathy. In: Cervero F, Bennett GJ, Headley PM, eds. Processing of sensory information in the superficial dorsal horn of the spinal cord. Amsterdam: Plenum Press; 1989: 463–471.
11. Dubner R, Ren K. Central mechanisms of thermal and mechanical hyperalgesia following tissue inflammation. In: Boivi J, Hansson P, Lindblom U, eds. Touch, temperature and pain in health and

disease: mechanisms and assessments, Vol. 3. Seattle: IASP Press; 1994: 267.

12. Wilcox GL. Excitatory neurotransmitters and pain. In: Bond MR, Charlton JE, Woolf CJ, eds. Proceedings on the 6th World Congress on Pain. Pain research and clinical management series, Vol. 4. Amsterdam: Elsevier; 1991: 97–117.

13. Siebert K, Zhang Y, Leahy K, et al. Pharmacological and biological demonstration of the role of cyclooxygenase 2 in inflammation and pain. Proc Natl Acad Sci USA 1994; 91: 12013–12017.

14. Walker JS. NSAID: an update on their analgesic effects. Clin Exp Pharmacol Physiol 1995; 22: 855–860.

15. Stein C. Peripheral mechanisms of opioid analgesia. Anesth Analg 1993; 76: 182–191.

16. Stein C, Millan MJ, Shippenberg TS, et al. Peripheral opioid receptors mediating antinociception in inflammation: evidence for involvement of mu, delta and kappa receptors. J Pharmacol Exp Ther 1989; 248: 1269–1275.

17. Aasbo V, Raeder JC, Grogaard B, et al. No additional analgesic effect of intraarticular morphine or bupivacaine compared with placebo after elective knee arthroscopy. Acta Anaesthesiol Scand 1996; 40: 585–588.

18. Devor M. The pathophysiology of damaged peripheral nerves. In: Wall PD, Melzack R, eds. Textbook of pain. 3rd edn. London: Churchill Livingstone; 1994: 79–100.

19. Backonja MM. Local anesthetics as adjuvant analgesics. J Pain Symptom Manage 1994; 9: 491–499.

20. Dahl JB, Moiniche S, Kehlet H. Wound infiltration with local anesthetics for postoperative pain relief [editorial]. Acta Anaesthiol Scand 1994; 38: 7–14.

21. Kissin I. Preemptive analgesia: why its effect is not always obvious. Anesthesiology 1996; 84: 1015–1019.

22. Katz J, Jackson M, Kavanagh BP, et al. Acute pain after thoracic surgery predicts long-term post-thoracotomy pain. Clin J Pain 1996; 12: 50–55.

23. Breivik H. Pre-emptive analgesia. Curr Opin Anesth 1994; 7: 458–461.

24. Bridenbaugh PO. Pre-emptive analgesia—is it clinically relevant? Anesth Analg 1994; 78: 203–204.

25. Pedersen JL, Crawford ME, Dahl JB, et al. Effect of pre-emptive nerve block on inflammation and hyperalgesia after human thermal injury. Anesthesiology 1996; 84: 1020–1026.

26. Hogan QH, Abram SE. Diagnostic and prognostic neural blockade. In: Cousins MJ, Bridenbaugh PO. Neural blockade in clinical anesthesia and management of pain. 3rd edn. Philadelphia: Lippincott-Raven; 1998: 837–877.

27. Tuominen M, Haasio J, Hekali R, et al. Continuous interscalene brachial plexus block: clinical efficacy, technical problems, and bupivacaine plasma concentrations. Acta Anaesthesiol Scand 1989; 33: 84–88.

28. Grant SA, Nielsen KC, Greengrass RA, et al. Continuous peripheral nerve block for ambulatory surgery. Reg Anesth Pain Med 2001;26: 209–214.

29. O'Driscoll SW, Giori NJ. Continuous passive motion (CPM): theory and principles of clinical application. J Rehabil Res Dev 2000; 37:179–188.

30. Taras JS, Behrman MJ. Continuous peripheral nerve block in replantation and revascularization. J Reconstr Microsurg 1998; 14: 17–21.

31. Sarma VJ. Long-term continuous axillary plexus blockade using 0.25% bupivacaine: a study of 3 cases. Acta Anaesthesiol Scand 1990; 34: 511–513.

32. Capdevila X, Barthelet Y, Biboulet PH, et al. Effects of perioperative analgesic technique on the surgical outcome and duration of rehabilitation after major knee surgery. Anesthesiology 1999; 91: 8–15.

33. Gaumann DM, Lennon RL, Wedel DJ. Continuous axillary block for postoperative pain management. Reg Anesth 1988; 13: 77–82.

34. Bergman BD, Hebl JR, Kent J, et al. Neurologic complications of 405 consecutive continuous axillary catheters. Anesth Analg 2003; 96: 247–252.

35. Brown DL, Ransom DM, Hall JA, et al. Regional anesthesia and local anesthetic–induced systemic toxicity: seizure frequency and accompanying cardiovascular changes. Anesth Analg 1995: 81: 321–328.

36. Horlocker TT, Kufner RP, Bishop AT, et al. The risk of persistent paresthesia is not increased with repeated axillary block. Anesth Analg 1999; 88: 382–387.

37. Cheng SL, Morrey BF. Treatment of the mobile, painful arthritic elbow by distraction interposition arthroplasty. J Bone Joint Surg Br 2000; 82: 233–238.

38. Horlocker TT. Regional anesthesia in the anticoagulated patient: defining the risks. The Second ASRA Consensus Conference on Neuraxial Anesthesia and Anticoagulation. Reg Anesth Pain Med 2003; 28: 172–197.

39. Horlocker TT, Wedel DJ, Benzun H et al. Regional Anesthesia in the anticoagulated patient: defining the risks. (The second ASRA consensus conference on neuraxial anesthesia and anticoagulation). Reg Anesthesia Pain Med 2003; 28: 172–197.

40. Cooke ED. Monitoring during low-dose heparin prophylaxis. N Engl J Med 1976; 294: 1066–1067.

41. Farrar MD, Scheybani M, Nolte H. Upper extremity block effectiveness and complications. Reg Anesth 1981; 6: 133–134.

42. Urmey WF, Talts KH, Sharrock ME. One hundred percent incidence of hemidiaphragmatic paresis associated with interscalene brachial plexus anesthesia diagnosed by ultrasonography. Anesth Analg 1991; 73: 498–503.

43. Pere P, Pitkanen M, Rosenberg P. Effect of continuous interscalene brachial plexus block on diaphragm motion and on ventilatory function. Acta Anaesthesiol Scand 1992: 36: 53–57.

44. Urmey WF, McDonald M. Hemidiaphragmatic paresis during interscalene brachial plexus block: effect on pulmonary function and chest wall mechanics. Anesth Analg 1992; 74: 352–357.

45. McIntyre JWR. Regional anesthesia safety. In: Finucane BT, ed. Complications of regional anesthesia. Philadelphia: Churchill-Livingstone; 1999: 1–30.

46. Brand L, Papper EM. A comparison of supraclavicular and axillary techniques for brachial plexus blocks. Anesthesiology 1961; 22:226–229.

47. De Jong RH. Local anesthetics adverse effects. In: Chambers C, ed. Local anesthetics. Springfield, IL: Charles C Thomas; 1977: 254.

48. Casey WF. Respiratory failure following intercostal nerve blockade. Anaesthesia 1984; 39: 351–354.

49. Cory PC, Mulroy MF. Postoperative respiratory failure following intercostal block. Anesthesiology 1981; 54: 418–419.

50. Bamford C, Sibley W, Laguna J. Anesthesia in multiple sclerosis. Can J Neurol Sci 1978; 5: 41–44.

51. Schapira K. Is lumbar puncture harmful in multiple sclerosis? J Neurol Neurosurg Psychiatr 1959; 22: 238.

52. Kochi T, Oka T, Mizuguchi T. Epidural anesthesia for patients with amyotrophic lateral sclerosis. Anesth Analg 1989; 68: 410–412.

53. Leventhal SR, Orkin FK, Hirsch RA. Prediction of the need for postoperative mechanical ventilation in myasthenia gravis. Anesthesiology 1980; 53: 26–30.

54. McGrady EM. Management of labour and delivery in a patient with Guillain–Barré syndrome. Anaesthesia 1987; 42: 899.

55. Romano E, Gullo A. Hypoglycemic coma following epidural analgesia. Anaesthesia 1980; 35: 1084–1086.

CHAPTER 5

Complications, toxicity, and safety

COMPLICATIONS AND TOXICITY

Principles underlying complications and errors

A complication is an undesirable, *unexpected* event occurring in the course of an intervention. It is necessary to differentiate between such events and the side effects one can normally expect to encounter in clinical practice. Side effects, in general, are predictable occurrences, and their prompt recognition and treatment can avoid more serious sequelae. Complications, on the other hand, may occur as a result of human factors on the part of the anesthesiologist, be attributable to environmental or equipment factors, or occur secondary to 'system' factors.

Human factors can be defined as lapses in or lack of safe habit, or the occurrence of a vigilance decrement resulting from sleep deprivation, fatigue, recent alcohol or drug ingestion, or boredom. Inexperience on the part of the anesthesiologist is likely to contribute to poor decision-making or an error in judgment. An important component in the avoidance of complications arising from these factors is awareness of anesthesiologists as individuals and of their role in complication development. They should thus seek to establish safe working practices and individual self-discipline that may act to counterbalance these risks.[1-3]

Environmental factors leading to complications may include lack of appropriate patient-monitoring systems and protocols, inadequate drug identification systems, or pressures originating from practice managers, surgeons, or financial concerns.

Patient selection and management are dealt with briefly in this chapter. Selection of an anesthetic technique that fits the patient, surgeon, and anesthesiologist at a particular point in time will form the basis of a successful intervention.

Systemic toxicity of local anesthetic drugs

Toxic reactions following local anesthetic drug administration can involve the CNS and/or the cardiovascular system. CNS toxicity is more common, occurs in association with lesser plasma drug concentrations, and responds more readily to treatment.

Central nervous system toxicity

The signs and symptoms of local anesthetic–induced CNS toxicity are shown in Fig. 5.1. An initial phase of CNS excitability, as demonstrated by light-headedness, dizziness, visual and auditory disturbance, muscle twitching, and convulsions, is followed by CNS depression, with coma then respiratory depression and arrest. This sequence of events occurs because of an initial inhibition, at lower concentrations, of inhibitory pathways in the amygdala. At greater concentrations, both inhibitory and excitatory pathways are inhibited, resulting in generalized CNS depression.[5-8]

The toxic potential of each anesthetic drug is related to its potency as an anesthetic agent (Table 5.1),[9] and the rate at which it is injected or absorbed (Fig. 5.2). Hypercapnia and acidosis lower the convulsive threshold for local anesthetic drugs. This occurs in a number of ways. A high pCO_2 will increase cerebral blood flow, resulting in higher rates of drug delivery; decreased intracellular pH facilitates the formation of

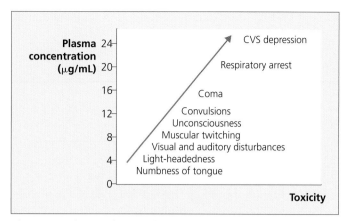

Figure 5.1 Relations of signs and symptoms of local anesthetic toxicity to plasma concentrations of lidocaine.
(From Covino BG, Wildsmith JAW. Clinical Pharmacology of Local Anesthetic Agents. In Cousins MJ, Bridenbaugh PO (eds). Neural Blockade in Clinical Anesthesia and Management of Pain, 3rd edn. Philadelphia: © Lippincott-Raven; 1998.)

Agent	CD (mg/kg)		
	pCO_2 25–40 mmHg	pCO_2 65–81 mmHg	Change in CD_{100}
Procaine	35	17	51
Mepivacaine	18	10	44
Prilocaine	22	12	45
Lidocaine	15	7	53
Bupivacine	5	2.5	50

(From Covino BG, Wildsmith JAW. Clinical Pharmacology of Local Anesthetic Agents. In Cousins MJ, Bridenbaugh PO (eds). Neural Blockade in Clinical Anesthesia and Management of Pain, 3rd edn. Philadelphia: © Lippincott-Raven; 1998.)

Table 5.1 Effect of pCO_2 on the convulsive threshold (CD_{100}) of various local anesthetics in cats.

the cationic form of drug, i.e. the active form; and hypercapnia and acidosis result in diminished protein-binding of drug, thereby making available a greater proportion of free drug.[10]

Local anesthetic–induced seizures are effectively terminated with barbiturate or benzodiazepine drugs.[11,12] The doses required are small and one should remain mindful that their myocardial depressant effects are additive to those of local anesthetic drugs.

Cardiovascular system toxicity

The depolarization phase of the action potential in cardiac tissue differs from nerve tissue in that the fast influx of Na^+ is followed by a slow influx of Ca^{2+}. This influx of Ca^{2+} is responsible for the spontaneous depolarization that is characteristic of cardiac tissue (Fig. 5.3, Table 5.2). Local anesthetic drugs

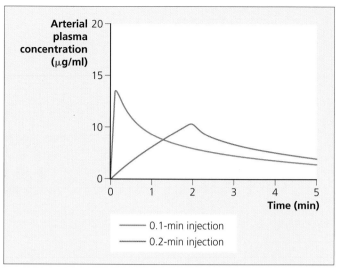

Figure 5.2 Arterial plasma concentrations following intravenous injection of 100 mg of lidocaine hydrochloride over 0.1 and 2 min to simulate concentrations of an inadvertant intravenous injection during a block procedure. Prolonging injection time reduces peak concentrations.
(From Covino BG, Wildsmith JAW. Clinical Pharmacology of Local Anesthetic Agents. In Cousins MJ, Bridenbaugh PO (eds). Neural Blockade in Clinical Anesthesia and Management of Pain, 3rd edn. Philadelphia: © Lippincott-Raven; 1998.)

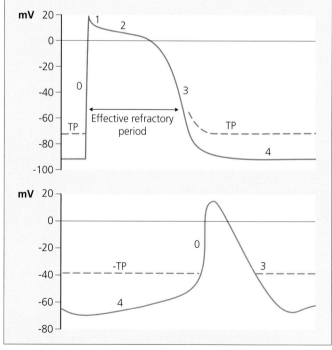

Figure 5.3 Cardiac action potential recorded from a ventricular contractile cell (**A**) or atrial pacemaker cell. (**B**) TP, threshold potential.
(From Stoelting RK. Heart. In: Pharmacology and physiology in anesthetic practice. 2nd ed. Philadelphia: © JB Lippincott; 1991.)

Phase	Ion	Movement across cell membrane
0	Na^+	In
1	K^+	Out
	Cl^-	In
2	Ca^{2+}	In
	K^+	Out
3	K^+	Out
4	Na^+	In

(From Stoelting RK. Heart. In: Pharmacology and physiology in anesthetic practice. 2nd ed. Philadelphia: © JB Lippincott; 1991.)

Table 5.2 Ion movement during phases of the cardiac action potential

depress the maximal depolarization rate of the cardiac action potential, V_{max}, secondary to inhibition of Na^+ conductance. With increasing concentrations of local anesthetics, prolongation of conduction times occurs, producing an increase in the P–R interval and QRS duration. At greater concentrations this is followed by sinus bradycardia, sinus arrest, and atrioventricular dissociation.[14,15] Local anesthetics also profoundly depress cardiac contractility, a phenomenon that may be related to the displacement of Ca^{2+} from the sarcolemma.[16–18]

The CC/CNS ratio is that of the dosage required for cardiovascular collapse (CC) to the dosage required to produce convulsions. It is approximately 7.1 for lidocaine and 3.7 for bupivacaine, suggesting a greater margin of safety in the use of lidocaine.[19] The high lipid-solubility of bupivacaine results in a slow rate of dissociation from the tissues, and thus a persistent effect on V_{max}. Cardiovascular collapse resulting from bupivacaine is therefore resistant to treatment. The potential for cardiac toxicity is enhanced in pregnancy, for reasons not fully understood, and also in the presence of hypoxia and hypercapnia.[20–22] These factors enhance the toxic potential of bupivacaine to a greater degree than they do lidocaine.

Peripheral vasculature

Local anesthetic drugs have a biphasic action on vascular smooth muscle.[23] At low concentrations they produce vasoconstriction. As the concentration increases, the effect becomes one of vasodilatation. These observations have been explained as being due to stimulation of spontaneous myogenic activity at low concentrations and inhibition of the same at greater concentrations.

Following an inadvertent intravascular injection of an amide local anesthetic, should the plasma concentration reach levels sufficient to produce CNS toxicity, one may also observe an increase in blood pressure, heart rate, and cardiac output. As the plasma concentration increases, reversible cardiovascular depression ensues, associated with a decrease in cardiac output and systemic blood pressure. Finally, myocardial contractility becomes profoundly depressed, marked peripheral vasodilatation occurs, and cardiac arrest ensues.

Nerve injury

Nerve stimulation is the technique of choice for locating a peripheral nerve. Prospective studies have demonstrated that a paresthesia technique can significantly increase the risk of postblock neuropathies (2.8%), while the transarterial approach to the brachial plexus is associated with paresthesia in as many as 40% of cases,[24,25] producing neuropathy in 0.8% (Table 5.3). In contrast, a nerve stimulation technique aims to avoid nerve contact and has been shown to produce important block-related neuropathies in only 0–0.3% of cases.[27]

The risk of penetrating a nerve fascicle is reduced when a short-bevel (45°) needle is used compared with a standard long-bevel (15°) needle, the reason being that nerve fascicles tend to roll away more readily from the advancing short-bevel needle tip.[28] Although the incidence of injury is less with short-bevel needles, when injury does occur it is more severe.

Intraneural needle position is associated with painful paresthesias on injection, and intraneural injection causes nerve damage and cell death by mechanical disruption, disruption of the blood–nerve barrier, high endoneural pressure (above capillary perfusion pressure) (Fig. 5.4), and direct neurotoxicity of local anesthetic agent. This situation is further aggravated if the solution contains epinephrine.[29,30] Therefore it is important to maintain verbal contact with the patient, avoid paresthesias, administer small incremental doses of drug, and reposition the needle if paresthesias are elicited.

In attempting to establish the etiology of nerve lesions in the postoperative period, the differential diagnosis must initially take into account patient positioning, tourniquet use, surgical trauma, and the presence of tight casts or dressings.[31–33] Follow-up of the patient in the immediate postoperative period will help to avoid inaccurate labeling of the deficit as 'anesthesia-related'.

Allergic reactions

Allergic reactions to local anesthetics occur rarely.[34] Indeed, most 'allergic reactions' to local anesthetics are in fact adverse reactions. Nevertheless, *para*-aminobenzoic acid is a product of the hydrolysis of ester local anesthetics and is a known allergen.[35–37] Allergy to amide local anesthetics is still rarer. However, some preparations contain methylparaben (an allergen), because of its excellent bacteriostatic and fungistatic properties.[38] After a case of allergy to a local anesthetic agent, intradermal testing of the full range of anesthetic agents is worthwhile, because allergy to one agent does not necessarily imply allergy to another.[37,39]

Reference	Block	No. of cases	Neural complications (%)
Bonica et al (1949)[64]	Supraclavicular plexus	1100	0
Moberg & Dhunér (1951)[65]	Supraclavicular plexus	300	5.7
Woolley & Vandam (1959)[66]	Supraclavicular plexus	106	7.5
Brand & Papper (1961)[67]	Supraclavicular plexus	230	2.2
Schmidt et al (1981)[68]	Supraclavicular plexus	342	0.9
Brand & Papper (1961)[69]	Axillary	246	0.8
De Jong (1961)[70]	Axillary	94	1.1
Hamelberg et al (1962)[71]	Axillary	250	1.2
Wall (1975)[72]	Axillary	431	0.2
Moore et al (1978)[73]	Axillary and plexus	652	0
Selander et al (1979)[74]	Axillary paresthesia	290	2.8
	Axillary, no paresthesia	243	0.8
Plevak et al (1983)[75]	Axillary paresthesia	477	2.9
	Axillary transarterial	239	0.8
Winchell & Wolfe (1985)[76]	Axillary	816	0.4
Tourtier et al (1989)[77]	Axillary paresthesia	758	0.9
	Axillary transarterial	642	0.3
Davis et al (1991)[78]	Axillary	530	0
Stan et al (1995)[79]	Axillary transarterial	1000	0.2
Löfström et al (1966)[80]	Intraulnar	25	12
Mogensen & Mattsson (1980)[81]	Intramedian	53	7.5

*Note the higher frequency of postblock neuropathies with paresthesia technique, which was also used for supraclavicular blocks and after intraneural blocks.
(From Selander D. Peripheral Nerve Injury after Regional Anesthesia. In Finucane, BT (Ed). Complications of Regional Anesthesia. Philadelphia, Churchill Livingstone, 1999, with permission from the American Society of Regional Anesthesia and Pain Medicine.)

Table 5.3. Survey of reported neuropathies after upper extremity block*

Infection

The presence of infection at the site of puncture is generally accepted as being a contraindication to regional anesthesia. The paucity of reports detailing infective complications of peripheral nerve block suggests that local and generalized infections following nerve blocks are rare. Disastrous infective complications continue to be reported following central neuraxial block, however, and the increasing use of peripheral nerve catheters suggests some elementary precautions be taken in this regard.[40] Unfortunately, no recommendations exist as to aseptic technique for spinal, epidural, or peripheral nerve block.[41] A review of the literature serves to highlight the following points:[40]

- The combined use of cap and mask should be encouraged for the duration of the procedure. Caps should be required of the patient also.[42–47]
- Long-sleeved sterile gowns should be used for catheter techniques.[48]
- Effective hand-washing is the single most cost-effective part of any aseptic techniques. Only nails and subungual regions should be brushed.[49]
- Chlorhexidine and polyvinylpyrrolidone-iodine (PVPI) are equally effective.[50]
- Hand-washing must precede the donning of sterile gloves, because microperforations can occur.
- The European Committee for Standardization recommends 60% isopropanol, in two portions of 3 mL each applied as a hand-rub for 60 s, as the most effective method of reducing bacteria. No solution is sporicidal.[51]
- The American Society of Anesthesiologists recommends PVPI, chlorhexidine, iodine tincture, or ethanol 70% for skin asepsis. A skin contact period of at least 2 min is required for any to be effective.[52]
- Chlorhexidine appears to have a more prolonged effect and should be used when an indwelling catheter is inserted.[53]

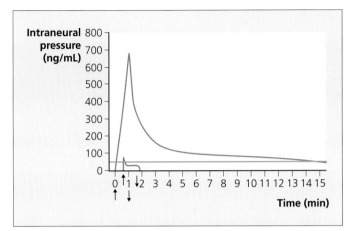

Figure 5.4 Recordings of intraneural pressure during and after injection of 100 μL in the sciatic nerve of a rabbit using an injection pump. Note the slow pressure decrease after intrafascicular injection. Green line, intrafascicular injection; blue line, epineural injection; arrows, start and end of injection; orange line, estimated endoneural capillary perfusion pressure. (From Selander D. Peripheral Nerve Injury after Regional Anesthesia. In Finucane, BT (Ed). Complications of Regional Anesthesia. Philadelphia, Churchill Livingstone, 1999, with permission from the American Society of Regional Anesthesia and Pain Medicine.)

■ When aspirating drugs from non-sterile ampoules, a 0.2-μm filter should be used to avoid contamination from small glass fragments, and the ampoules should be wiped with alcohol before opening.[54]

Neural toxicity of local anesthetics

All clinically used local anesthetic agents are potentially toxic at high concentrations. Under normal conditions, the drug is rapidly diluted and absorbed. However, if the nerve is ischemic or the drug is injected intraneurally, the nerve is exposed to greater than normal concentrations of local anesthetic and for a longer than expected period of time. This situation is exacerbated with epinephrine-containing solutions.[55] Lidocaine was shown to have a greater neurotoxic potential in this regard than the other clinically used agents.

Myotoxicity of local anesthetics

Injection of local anesthetic into muscle results in focal necrosis; the more potent the agent, the greater the degree of injury that results. This effect is localized and regeneration has been shown to be complete within 2 weeks. The changes are of a subclinical nature and do not appear to contribute to the perioperative morbidity of regional anesthesia.[56] Some concern has been raised, however, regarding the role of local anesthetic drugs in the development of diplopia following cataract surgery performed under regional anesthesia. A 0.25% incidence of diplopia related to anesthetic factors has

been reported.[57] It appears to be more common following peribulbar block than retrobulbar block and does not occur following topical or general anesthesia. The inferior rectus muscle is typically involved following infraorbital injection. Possible mechanisms underlying this complication are direct muscle injury from the block needle, vascular compromise secondary to elevated local pressures, and myotoxicity of the local anesthetic.

SAFE CONDUCT OF REGIONAL ANESTHESIA

Patient selection

Appropriate patient selection for a regional anesthetic technique involves consideration of patient factors, the medical history, specific investigations, psychological preparation, the planned surgical intervention, and the expertise of the anesthesiologist.

When general anesthesia poses serious risks—for example in the patient with a full stomach, difficult airway, or poor general medical condition—regional anesthesia is quite often the anesthetic technique of choice. However, there are various medical conditions where the choice of anesthetic technique remains controversial. These include degenerative neurologic disease, diabetes, and severe cardiovascular and respiratory disease. These conditions are dealt with in more detail in Chapter 4. As for all patients, a thorough preanesthetic medical and laboratory evaluation is indicated in order to perform an appropriate risk–benefit analysis.

Morbid obesity, physical deformities, arthritis, fractures, local infection, or locally enlarged lymph glands may serve to hinder the administration of an adequate block and so should be noted prior to the formulation of an anesthetic plan. The disoriented or psychologically deranged patient may not only make intraoperative management difficult but render the safe performance of a block impossible. A history of concurrent medication, such as anticoagulants (Box 5.1) or vasoactive drugs, should also be taken into account because of the implications for the performance and administration of regional anesthesia (see Ch. 4).

The evaluation of the patient must also include systemic disease, current medications, previous anesthetics, allergies, state of dentition, and family history. Occasionally it may be necessary to convert a regional to a general anesthetic technique. Therefore all the information relevant to provision of general anesthesia should be obtained.

The patient interview allows one to obtain the relevant information outlined above; it is also an opportunity to prepare the patient psychologically for the procedure and the perioperative experience in general and to obtain informed consent. Informed consent implies that the material risks and

Box 5.1 Precautions for combined use of anticoagulants and neuraxial block

- Strict patient selection to exclude other possible bleeding diastheses.
- Perform regional anesthesia only when clotting variables are acceptable.
- Use atraumatic technique; if tap bloody, postpone surgery and perform under general anesthesia 24 h later.
- Full heparinization no sooner than 60 min after initiation of block.
- Monitor clotting times throughout and maintain $1\frac{1}{2}$–2 times baseline value; reverse heparin effect if necessary.
- Remove spinal or epidural catheters at least 120 min after stopping heparinization and with normal clotting time.
- Maintain strict neurologic surveillance.

(From Vandermeulen EP, VanAken H, Vermylen J: Anticoagulants and spinal-epidural anesthesia. Anesth Analg 1994; 79: 1165.)

Patient group	Solids and non-clear liquids†	Clear liquids
Adults	6–8 h or none after 12 midnight‡	2–3 h
Children > 36 months old	6–8 h	2–3 h
Children 6–36 months old	6 h	2–3 h
Children <6 months old	4–6 h	2 h

*Gastric emptying may be influenced by many factors including anxiety, pain, abnormal autonomic function (e.g. diabetes), pregnancy, and mechanical obstruction. Therefore the suggestions above do not guarantee that complete gastric emptying has occurred. Unless contraindicated, children should be offered clear liquids until 2–3 h before sedation to minimize the risk of dehydration.
†This includes milk, formula, and breast milk. (High fat content may delay gastric emptying.)
‡There are no data to establish whether a 6–8-h fast is equivalent to an overnight fast prior to sedation or analgesia.
(From the American Society of Anesthesiologists,[61] with permission of ASA.)

Table 5.4 Example of fasting protocol for sedation and analgesia for elective procedures*

benefits of the proposed procedure have been explained, as well as those of the available alternatives. When one explains the reasons for choosing one technique over another, and when appropriate assurances as to the standard of care are given, most patients will accept regional anesthesia. Assurances as to the availability of block supplementation and sedation up to the level of general anesthesia should be given, as well as a detailed description of the performance of the block(s). Patients may perceive sensations of an unusual or bizarre nature under regional anesthesia; therefore explanation, reassurance, and appropriate sedation should be provided. Most patients who have benefited from a well-executed regional anesthetic will choose the same technique for future interventions when possible.[59]

Preoperative fasting

Traditionally, adult patients scheduled for a surgical intervention were required to abstain from both oral solids and fluids for a minimum of 6 h, and, more often, from midnight the night before. However, unrestricted clear fluids (water and apple juice) up to 2 h before surgery have been shown to result

in no significant difference in mean residual gastric volume or pH.[60] As a consequence, a number of organizations have amended their fasting guidelines (Table 5.4).[61]

Equipment

In 1986, the Department of Anesthesia of Harvard Medical School published detailed, mandatory standards for minimal patient monitoring during anesthesia.[62] For the safe conduct of regional anesthesia, in addition to the presence of an anesthesiologist or nurse anesthetist, the following equipment should be available and used:

- pulse oximeter
- blood pressure monitor
- ECG monitor
- peripheral nerve stimulator.

The equipment included in Box 5.2 should also be available for immediate use, and a checklist performed prior to anesthesia. In addition, the nerve stimulator to be used should be checked according to the manufacturer's instructions prior to each use.

Box 5.2 Preanesthetic checklist

A. Gas pipelines
- Secure connections between terminal units (outlets) and anesthetic machine.

B. Anesthetic machine
1.
   - Turn on machine master switch and all other necessary electrical equipment.
   - Line oxygen (40–60 p.s.i., 275–415 kPa).
   - Line nitrous oxide (40–60 p.s.i., 275–415 kPa).
   - Adequate reserve cylinder oxygen pressure.
   - Adequate reserve cylinder nitrous oxide content.
   - Check for leaks and turn off cylinders.
   - Flow meter function of oxygen and nitrous oxide over the working range.
2.
   - Vaporizer filled.
   - Filling ports pin-indexed and closed.
   - Ensure 'on/off' function and turn off.
3. Functioning oxygen bypass (flush).
4. Functioning oxygen failsafe device.
5.
   - Oxygen analyzer calibrated and turned-on functioning mixer (where available).
   - Attempt to create a hypoxic O_2/N_2O mixture and verify correct changes in flow and/or alarm.
6. Functioning common fresh gas outlet.
7. Ventilator function verified.
8. Backup ventilation equipment available and functioning.

Note: If an anesthetist uses the same machine in successive cases, departmental policy may permit performing an abbreviated checklist between cases.

C. Breathing circuit
1. Correct assembly of circuit to be used.
2. Patient circuit connected to common fresh gas outlet.
3. Oxygen flow meter turned on.
4.
   - Check for exit of fresh gas at face mask.
   - Pressurize. Check for leaks and integrity at circuit (e.g. Pethick text for coaxial).
5. Functioning high-pressure relief valve.
6. Unidirectional valves and soda lime.
7. Functioning adjustable pressure relief valve.

D. Vacuum system
- Suction adequate.

E. Scavenging system
- Correctly connected to patient circuit and functioning.

F. Routine equipment
1.
   - Airway.
   - Functioning laryngoscope (backup available).
   - Appropriate tracheal tubes: patency of lumen and integrity of cuff.
   - Appropriate oropharyngeal airways.
   - Stylet.
   - Magill forceps.
2. I.v. supplies.
3. Blood pressure cuff of appropriate size.
4. Stethoscope.
5. ECG monitor.
6. Pulse oximeter.
7. Capnograph.
8. Temperature monitor.
9. Functioning low- and high-pressure alarm.

G. Drugs
1. Adequate supply of frequently used drugs and i.v. solutions.
2. Appropriate doses of drugs in labeled syringes.

H. Location of special equipment in each anesthetizing location
1. Defibrillators.
2. Emergency drugs.
3. Difficult intubation kit.

(From McIntyre JWR. Regional Anesthesia Safety. In Finucane BT (ed). Complications of Regional Anesthesia. Philadelphia, Churchill Livingstone, 1999, with permission from the American Society of Regional Anesthesia and Pain Medicine.)

References

1. Cooper JB, Gaba DM. A strategy for preventing accidents. Int. Anesthesiol Clin 1989; 27: 148–152.
2. Weinger MB, Englund CE. Ergonomic and human factors affecting anesthetic vigilance and monitoring performance in the operating room environment. Anesthesiology 1990; 73: 995–1021.
3. Gaba DM. Human error in anesthetic mishaps. Int Anesthesiol Clin 1989; 27: 137–147.
4. Covino BG, Wildsmith JAW. Clinical pharmacology of local anesthetic agents. In: Neural blockade in clinical anesthesia and management of pain. 3rd edn. Cousins MJ, Bridenbaugh PO, eds. Philadelphia: Lippincott-Raven; 1998: 97–128.
5. DeJong RH, Robles R, Corbin RW. Central actions of lidocaine—synaptic transmission. Anesthesiology 1969; 30: 19–23.
6. Huffman RD, Yim GKW. Effects of diphenylaminoethanol and lidocaine on central inhibition. Int J Neuropharmacol 1969; 8: 217–225.
7. Tanaka K, Yamasaki M. Blocking of cortical inhibitory synapses by intravenous lidocaine. Nature 1966; 209: 207–208
8. Wagman IH, DeJong RH, Prince DA. Effects of lidocaine on the central nervous system. Anesthesiology 1967; 28: 155–172.

9. Liu PL, Feldman HS, Giasi R, et al. Comparative CNS toxicity of lidocaine, etidocaine, bupivacaine and tetracaine in awake dogs following rapid IV administration. Anesth Analg 1983; 62: 375–379.
10. Englesson S. The influence of acid–base changes on central nervous system toxicity of local anesthetic agents. Acta Anaesthesiol Scand 1974; 18: 79–87.
11. Covino BG. Toxicity and systemic effects of local anesthetic agents. In: Strichartz G, ed. Local anesthetics, handbook of experimental pharmacology, Vol. 81. New York: Springer-Verlag; 1987: 187–209.
12. Davis NL, DeJong RH. Successful resuscitation following massive bupivacaine overdose. Anesth Analg 1982; 61: 62–64.
13. Stoelting RK. Heart. In: Pharmacology and physiology in anesthetic practice. 2nd edn. Philadelphia: JB Lippincott; 1991.
14. Lieberman NA, Harris RS, Katz RI, et al. The effects of lidocaine on the electrical and mechanical activity of the heart. Am J Cardiol 1968; 22: 375–380.
15. Sugimoto T, Schaal FS, Dunn NM, et al. Electrophysiological effects of lidocaine in awake dogs. J Pharmacol Exp Ther 1969; 166: 146–150.
16. Block A, Covino BG. Effect of local anesthetic agents on cardiac conduction and contractility. Reg Anesth 1981;6:55–61.
17. Feldman HS, Covino BG, Sage DJ. Direct chronotropic and inotropic effects of local anesthetic agents in isolated guinea pig atria. Reg Anesth 1982; 7: 149–156.
18. Josephson I, Sperelakis N. Local anesthetic blockade of Ca^{2+}-mediated action potentials in cardiac muscle. Eur J Pharmacol 1976; 40: 201–208.
19. Morishima HO, Pederson H, Finster M, et al. Is bupivacaine more cardiotoxic than lidocaine? Anesthesiology 1983; 59: A409.
20. Morishima HO, Pederson H, Finster M, et al. Bupivacaine toxicity in pregnant and nonpregnant ewes. Anesthesiology 1985; 63: 134–139.
21. Sage DJ, Feldman HS, Arthur GR, et al. Influence of lidocaine and bupivacaine on isolated guinea pig atria in the presence of acidosis and hypoxia. Anesth Analg 1984; 63: 1–7.
22. Thigpen JW, Kotelko DM, Shnider SM, et al. Bupivacaine cardiotoxicity in hypoxic-acidotic sheep. Anesthesiology 1983; 59: A204.
23. Blair MR. Cardiovascular pharmacology of local anesthetics. Br J Anaesth 1975; 47: 247–252.
24. Selander D, Edshage S, Wolff T. Paresthesiae or no paresthesiae? Nerve lesions after axillary blocks. Acta Anaesth Scand 1979; 23: 27–33.
25. Plevak DJ, Linstromberg JW, Danielsson DR. Paresthesia vs non-paresthesia—the axillary block. Anesthesiology 1983; 59: A216.
26. Selander D. Peripheral nerve injury after regional anesthesia. In: Finucane BT, ed. Complications of regional anesthesia. Philadelphia: Churchill Livingstone; 1999: 105–115.
27. Auroy Y, Benhamou D, Bargues L, et al. Major complications of regional anesthesia in France. The SOS regional anesthesia hotline service. Anesthesiology 2002; 97: 1274–1280.
28. Selander D, Dhuner KG, Lundborg G. Peripheral nerve injury due to injection needles used for regional anesthesia. Acta Anaesthesiol Scand 1977; 21: 182–188.
29. Selander D, Sjöstrand J. Longitudinal spread of intraneurally injected local anesthetics: an experimental study in the initial distribution following intraneural injections. Acta Anaesthesiol Scand 1978; 22: 622–634.
30. Selander D, Brattsand R, Lundborg G. Local anesthetics: importance of mode of application, concentration and adrenaline for the appearance of nerve lesions: an experimental study of axonal degeneration and barrier damage after intrafascicular injection or topical application of bupivacaine (Marcain). Acta Anaesthesiol Scand 1979; 23: 127–136.
31. Nicholson MJ, McAlpine FS. Neural injuries: association with surgical positions and operations. In: Martin JT, ed. Positioning in anesthesia and surgery. Philadelphia: WB Saunders; 1978: 193.
32. Winchell SW, Wolfe R. The incidence of neuropathy following upper extremity nerve blocks. Reg Anesth 1985; 10: 12–15.
33. Kroll DA, Caplan RA, Posner K, et al. Nerve injury associated with anesthesia. Anesthesiology 1990; 73: 202–207.
34. Adriani J. Reactions to local anesthetics. JAMA 1966; 196: 405–408.
35. Aldrete JA, Johnson DA. Evaluation of intracutaneous testing for investigation of allergy to local anesthetic agents. Anesth Analg 1970; 49: 173–183.
36. Incaudo G, Schatz M, Patterson R, et al. Administration of local anesthetics to patients with a history of prior adverse reaction. J Allergy Clin Immunol 1978; 61: 339–345.
37. Brown DT, Beamish D, Wildsmith JAW. Allergic reaction to an amide local anaesthetic. Br J Anaesth 1981; 53: 435–437.
38. Nagel JE, Fuscaldo JT, Fireman P. Paraben allergy. JAMA 1977; 237: 1594–1595.
39. Fisher M, Pennington JC. Allergy to local anaesthesia. Br J Anaesth 1982; 54: 893–894.
40. Videira RLR, Ruiz-Neto PP, Brandao Neto M. Post spinal meningitis and asepsis. Acta Anaesthesiol Scand 2002; 46: 639–646.
41. Sellors JE, Cyna AM, Simmons SW. Aseptic precautions for inserting an epidural catheter: a survey of obstetric anaesthetists. Anaesthesia 2002; 57: 593–596.
42. Lurie S, Feinstein M, Heifetz C, et al. Iatrogenic bacterial meningitis after spinal anesthesia for pain relief during labour [letter]. J Clin Anesth 1999; 11: 438–439.
43. Dolinski SY, Gerancher JC. Unmasked mischief [letter]. Anesth Analg 2001; 92: 279–281.
44. McLure HA, Mannam M, Talboys CA, et al. The effect of facial hair and sex on the dispersal of bacteria below a masked subject. Anaesthesia 2000; 55: 173–176.
45. Hubble MJ, Weale AE, Perez JV, et al. Clothing in laminar-flow operating theatres. J Hosp Infect 1996; 32: 1–7.
46. Rogers KB. An investigation into the efficiency of disposable face masks. J Clin Pathol 1980; 33: 1086–1091.
47. Panikkar KK, Yentis SM. Wearing of masks for obstetric regional anesthesia: a postal survey. Anaesthesia 1996; 51: 398–400.
48. Sleth JC. Evaluation des mesures d'asepsie lors de la realisation d'un catheterisme epidural et perception de son risque infectieux. Resultats d'une enquête en Languedoc-Roussilon. Ann Fr Anesth Reanim 1998; 17: 408–414.
49. Handwashing Liaison Group. Hand washing: a modest measure—with big effects. Br Med J 1999; 318: 686.
50. Mimoz O, Karim A, Mercat A, et al. Chlorhexidine compared with povidone iodine as skin prep before blood culture. Ann Int Med 1999; 131: 834–837.
51. Rotter ML. Hand washing and hand disinfection. In: Mayhall CG, ed. Hospital epidemiology and infection control. 2nd edn. Philadelphia: Lippincott Williams & Wilkins; 1999: 1339–1355.
52. American Society of Anesthesiologists. Recommendations for infection control for the practice of anesthesiology. 2nd edn. Park Ridge, IL: ASA; 1998: 10.
53. Kinirons B, Mimoz O, Lafendi L. Chlorhexidine versus povidone iodine in preventing colonization of continuous epidural catheters in children. A randomized controlled trial. Anesthesiology 2001; 94: 239–244.
54. Tunstall ME, MacLennan FM. Contamination of opioids during preparation for regional anaesthesia [letter]. Anaesthesia 1997; 52: 290.

55. Kroin JS, Penn RD, Levy FE, et al. Effect of repetitive lidocaine infusion on peripheral nerve. Exp Neurol 1986; 94: 166–173.

56. Libelius R Sonesson B, Stamenovic BA, et al. Denervation-like changes in skeletal muscle after treatment with a local anesthetic (Marcain). J Anat 1970; 106: 297–309.

57. Gómez-Arnau JI,Yangüela J, Gonzáles A, et al. Anaesthesia-related diplopia after cataract surgery. Br J Anaesth 2003; 90: 189–193.

58. Vandermeulen EP, VanAken H, Vermylen J. Anticoagulants and spinal-epidural anesthesia. Anesth Analg 1994; 79: 1165–1177.

59. Klein SM, Nielsen KC, Greengrass RA, et al. Ambulatory discharge after long-acting peripheral nerve blockade: 2382 blocks with ropivacaine. Anesth Analg 2002; 94: 65–70.

60. Phillips S, Hutchinson S, Davidson T. Preoperative drinking does not affect gastric contents. Br J Anaesth 1993; 70: 6–9.

61. American Society of Anesthesiologists. Guidelines for sedation and analgesia by non-anesthesiologists. Park Ridge, IL: ASA; 1999: 3–11.

62. Eichhorn JH, Cooper JB, Cullen DJ. Standards for patient monitoring during anesthesia at Harvard Medical School. JAMA 1986; 256: 1017–1020.

63. McIntyre JWR. Regional anesthesia safety. In: Finucane BT, ed. Complications of regional anesthesia. Philadelphia: Churchill Livingstone; 1999: 1–30.

64. Bonica JJ, Moore DC, Orlov M. Brachial plexus block anesthesia. Am J Surg 1949; 78: 65

65. Moberg E, Dhunér K-G. Brachial plexus block analgesia with xylocaine. J Bone Joint Surg. 1951; 33A: 884

66. Wooley EJ, Vandam LD. Neurological sequelae of brachial plexus nerve block. Ann Surg. 1959; 149: 53–60

67. Brand L, Papper EM. A comparison of supraclavicular and axillary techniques for brachial plexus blocks. Anesthesiology. 1961; 22: 226–229

68. Schmidt E, Racenberg E, Hilderbrand G et al. Komplikationen und gefahren der plexus-brachialis-anästhesie unter besonderer Berücksichtiging von Langzeitschaden. Anästh Intensivther Notfallmed. 1981; 16: 346–349

69. Brand L, Papper EM. A comparison of supraclavicular and axillary techniques for brachial plexus blocks. Anesthesiology. 1961; 22: 226–229

70. De Jong RH. Axillary block of the brachial plexus. Anesthesiology 1961; 22: 215–225

71. Hamelberg W, Dysart R, Bosomworth P. Perivascular axillary versus supraclavicular brachial plexus block and general anesthesia. Anesth Analg. 1962; 41; 85–90

72. Wall JJ. Axillary nerve blocks. Ann Surg.1959; 149: 53

73. Moore DC, Bridenbaugh LD, Thompson GE et al. Bupivacaine: a review of 11,080 cases. Anesth Analg. 1978: 57: 42–53

74. Selander D, Edshage S, Wolff T. Parasthesiae or no parasthesiae? Nerve lesions after axillary blocks. Acta Anaesth Scand. 1979; 23: 27–33

75. Plevak DJ, Linstromberg JW, Danielsson DR. Paresthesiae vs non-paresthesiae – the axillary block. Anesthesiology. 1983; 59: A216

76. Winchell SW, Wolfe R. The incidence of neuropathy following upper extremity nerve blocks. Reg Anesth 1985; 10: 12–15

77. Tourtier Y, Rébillion M, Delort J et al. Complications of axillary block using two techniques: experience with 1400 cases. Anesthesiology 1989; 71: A726

78. Davis WJ, Lennon RL, Wedel DJ. Brachial plexus anesthesia for outpatient surgical procedures on an upper extremity. Moyo Clinic Proc. 1991: 66: 544–547

79. Stan TC, Krantz MA, Solomon DL et al. The incidence of neurovascular complications following axillary brachial plexus block using a transarterial approach. Reg Anesth. 1995; 20: 486–492

80. Löfström B, Wennberg A, Widén L. Late disturbances in nerve function after block with local anesthetic agents. Acta Anesth Scand. 1966; 10: 111–122

81. Mogensen BA, Mattsson HS. Posttraumatic instability of the metacarpophalyngeal joint of the thumb. Hand. 1980; 12: 85–90

CHAPTER 6
Peripheral nerve block materials

NERVE STIMULATORS

In 1911, Stoffel demonstrated how a galvanic current could be applied to identify nerve fibers.[1] A year later, Perthes described how the use of electrical stimulation could improve the safety of neural block in the practice of anesthesia.[2]

Nerve stimulation is a popular technique for the location and identification of nerve fibers, particularly in Europe.[3] It was introduced into contemporary practice in 1973 by Montgomery and Raj against considerable opposition, particularly in the USA, where many practitioners advocated the dictum 'no paresthesia, no anesthesia'.[4,5] Nerve stimulation, through the intentional avoidance of direct contact with the nerve fiber, aims to reduce the risk of neurologic complications. However, the relations between stimulating current, motor and sensory responses, success rates, and needle–nerve distances are far from clear in the clinical setting.[6-8] The nerve stimulation method produces peripheral nerve injury in up to three cases in 10 000.[9] In contrast, the transarterial approach to brachial plexus anesthesia produces nerve lesions in 0.8% of cases and the paresthesia approach in 2.8%.[10,11] The following is a discussion on the theoretical as well as practical aspects of nerve stimulation and the equipment commonly used to locate nerves. The reader should remain cognizant of the fact that no definitive study outlining the exact nature of the relation between the stimulating current and the observed responses in clinical practice exists to date.

ELECTROPHYSIOLOGY

The electrochemical nature of nerve fiber conduction renders it amenable to electrical stimulation. The strength–duration curve demonstrates the relation between the intensity and duration of current in peripheral nerve stimulation (Fig. 6.1).

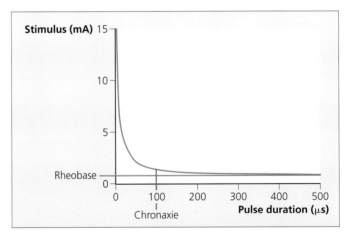

Figure 6.1 Strength–duration curve, cat sciatic nerve. The rheobase is the smallest current to stimulate the nerve with a long pulse width. The chronaxie is the pulse duration at a stimulus strength twice the rheobase. The curve was obtained from a cat sciatic nerve with the stimulating needle touching the nerve.
(From Pither C, Prithvi R, Ford D. The use of peripheral nerve stimulators for regional anesthesia. A review of experimental characteristics, techniques and clinical applications. Reg Anesth 1985; 10; 49–58, with permission from the American Society of Regional Anesthesia and Pain Medicine.)

43

The total charge applied to the nerve is a product of the current intensity and the duration of the pulse. The minimum in vitro quantity of current necessary to generate an action potential can be calculated from the equation

$$I = Ir (1 + C/t).$$

I is the current required, Ir the rheobase, C the chronaxie, and t the duration of stimulus. The rheobase is the minimum current required to depolarize a nerve when applied for a long period. The chronaxie is the duration of impulse necessary to stimulate at twice the rheobase.

The chronaxie of a motor nerve is less than that of a sensory nerve. In the clinical setting, therefore, a motor response may be elicited without stimulating pain fibers if the duration of impulse is short. Sensory nerves may also be identified using a nerve stimulator if the pulse duration is greater than $400 \, \mu s$ (Table 6.1).

Coulomb's law,

$$E = K (Q/r^2),$$

governs the relation between the stimulus intensity and the distance from the nerve. E is the current required, K a constant, Q the minimal current, and r the distance. The significance lies in the squaring of the distance. While one may thus approach the nerve through the progressive diminution of current, at distances greater than 0.5 cm from the nerve large currents are required; at greater than 2 cm, currents of up to 50 mA may be generated. These currents produce pain locally and require that appropriate care be taken in patients with intracardiac electrodes (Table 6.2).

Ohm's law describes the relation between potential difference (U), resistance (R), and intensity (I):

$$U = R \times I.$$

In practice, U corresponds to the potential difference between the poles of the nerve stimulator; R corresponds to the internal resistance of the patient and the resistance of the cables. The negative electrode is connected to the needle and the positive to the patient's skin via a gel electrode. Because the interior of

	Nerve fiber type	Chronaxie
Cat sural nerve	Aα	50–100 μs[13]
	Aδ	170 μs[14]
Cat saphenous nerve	C	400 μs[15]

(From Pither C, Prithvi R, Ford D. The use of peripheral nerve stimulators for regional anesthesia. A review of experimental characteristics, techniques and clinical applications. Reg Anesth 1985; 10; 49–58, with permission from the American Society of Regional Anesthesia and Pain Medicine.)

Table 6.1 Chronaxies of mammalian peripheral nerves

	On nerve	Distance (cm)		
		0.5	1	2
Stimulus	0.1	2.5	10	40
Current*	0.5	12.5	50	200
mA	1.0	25.0	100	400

*Current increases to unacceptable levels at distances greater than 2 cm.
(From Pither C, Prithvi R, Ford D. The use of peripheral nerve stimulators for regional anesthesia. A review of experimental characteristics, techniques and clinical applications. Reg Anesth 1985; 10; 49–58, with permission from the American Society of Regional Anesthesia and Pain Medicine.)

Table 6.2 Calculated values for current required to stimulate nerve at various distances from the nerve

Anodal vs. cathodal current required to stimulate peripheral nerve	Reference
× 4.57	BeMent & Ranck, 1969[16]
× 4.3	Ford et al, 1984[17]

(From Pither C, Prithvi R, Ford D. the use of peripheral nerve stimulators for regional anesthesia. A review of experimental characteristics, techniques and clinical applications. Reg Anesth 1985; 10; 49–58, with permission from the American Society of Regional Anesthesia and Pain Medicine.)

Table 6.3 Polarity of stimulation

a nerve at rest is negatively charged relative to the exterior, if the poles are reversed hyperpolarization of the nerve occurs; it is then necessary to apply a current of greater intensity to achieve the same motor response. These currents may be uncomfortable for the patient (Fig. 6.2, Table 6.3).

CHARACTERISTICS

The characteristics considered desirable in a nerve stimulator are constant current output; digital display; square-shaped, monophasic, negative impulse; variable output control; linear output; clearly marked polarity; short pulse width; variable stimulation frequency of 1 or 2 Hz; high-quality cables and connections; and indicators of power failure, circuit closure, high circuit resistance, and device malfunction.[17,18]

The resistance of the human body, cables, connections, etc., may vary between 1000 and 20 000 ohms. It is important that the current should not vary with these changes in resistance, i.e. the device should have a constant current output. As $U = R \times I$ (U being the potential difference between the poles of the

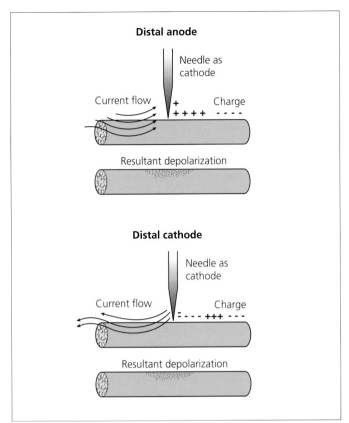

Figure 6.2 Preferential cathodal stimulation. With the needle as the cathode (**A**), electron flow is toward the needle, causing an area of depolarization around the needle tip. With the needle as anode (**B**), the area adjacent to the nerve is hypopolarized, with a zone of depolarization in a ring distant to the needle, an arrangement that requires more current to stimulate the nerve.
(From Pither C, Prithvi R, Ford D. The use of peripheral nerve stimulators for regional anesthesia. A review of experimental characteristics, techniques and clinical applications. Reg Anesth 1985; 10; 49–58, with permission from the American Society of Regional Anesthesia and Pain Medicine.)

device, R the impedance of the external electrical circuit, and I the current intensity), the nerve stimulator must be able to deliver a high output load to avoid a possible 20-fold change in the current delivered.

A digital display of the current intensity delivered is important as one approaches the nerve with very small currents. Knowledge of the precise intensity is vital for accurate nerve location. A final current intensity of 0.5 mA or less is associated with a high success rate in brachial plexus anesthesia.[19]

The current impulse needs to be square-shaped, monophasic, and negative. The amplitude corresponds to the intensity of the electric current and is expressed in milliamperes (mA); the duration is measured in ms or μs. It is important to have a short ascent and descent time to the impulse because the charge applied to the nerve is a product of the current and the duration. Therefore the more square-shaped the signal, the greater the precision of the instrument.

To be able to choose between several pulse widths is equally of value. A short pulse width of 50–100 μs is necessary because this corresponds to the chronaxies of mammalian Aδ fibers (see Table 6.1). According to Coulomb's law, the electrical field produced for a current intensity of constant duration is inversely proportional to the square of the distance:

$$E = K (Q/r^2)$$

(see previous section, *Electrophysiology*). Therefore one may bring the needle tip closer to the nerve through the progressive diminution of current intensity. Conversely, as one moves away from the nerve, currents of high intensity are required to stimulate the nerve.

The nerve stimulator should have a variable output control that operates on a linear scale. This means that the output of the device alters in proportion to the movement of the dial.

The negative lead must be attached to the needle for reasons already outlined. By convention, the negative lead is colored black and the positive red. To avoid confusion, clear labeling or non-interchangeable connections are required.

NEEDLES USED IN PERIPHERAL NERVE BLOCK

The needles used in nerve stimulation have been traditionally classified depending on whether or not they possess an insulating coat. Uninsulated needles are cheaper and may be less painful on insertion. However, the current emanates from the whole of the needle shaft, with the maximum current density just proximal to the tip. The needle is therefore still capable of eliciting a response when the tip has bypassed the nerve. Furthermore, as the current is widely dispersed through the length of the needle, a greater current intensity is required to generate the same electrical charge at the nerve for any given duration of impulse.

Insulated needles have high precision in locating nerves. The stimulating current is concentrated in, directed from, and forms a sphere around the needle tip. This is more likely to result in accurate delivery of local anesthetic solution. These needles are relatively expensive and skin puncture tends to be more difficult and uncomfortable for the patient. This group of needles may be further subdivided into those with a coated or an uncoated bevel. Needles with a coated bevel have the stimulating current more densely concentrated at the needle tip, resulting in more precision and the requirement for less current to stimulate the nerve (Figs 6.3, 6.4).[20]

PERIPHERAL NERVE CATHETERS

The first use of peripheral nerve catheters in the management of acute and chronic pain was described in 1946.[22] Initially,

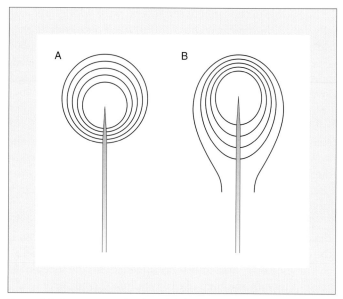

Figure 6.3 Computer-simulated models for zones of current density around the tips of insulated and uninsulated needles. The center of B is just proximal to the needle tip and most of the zone extends up the needle shaft. (From Bashein et al 1984,[20] with permission.)

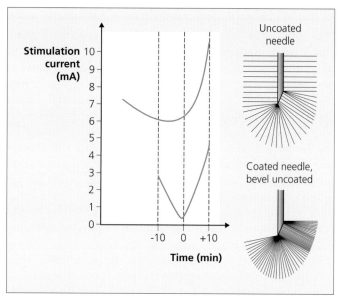

Figure 6.4 Comparison of current required to stimulate nerve against distance from nerve for various needle types.
(From B. Braun Medical Inc. Technical aspects of peripheral electrical nerve stimulation. Available: http://www.bbraunusa.com/stimuplex/pens1.html)

ureteral lacquered silk catheters were used. Developments in material technology have now provided us with nylon, polyurethane, and Teflon® catheters of high quality. These modern catheters are packaged with an appropriately sized stimulating short bevel or Tuohy needle. For example, an 18-G needle will accompany a 20-G catheter.

Catheters used for continuous peripheral nerve block need to be relatively stiff and blunt. This is in contrast to those used for neuraxial block, which need to be pliable and resistant to kinking and knotting. While nylon catheters may be degraded by phenol and ethanol, this problem does not occur with Teflon® catheters. Fortunately, local anesthetics appear to have no such degrading effects.[23]

Catheters capable of nerve stimulation have been marketed.[24] These devices may result in higher success rates in catheter placement; as with the current systems of advancing the catheter through or over the block needle, the relation between final catheter tip position and the stimulating needle tip position is often far from clear.

ULTRASOUND IN THE PRACTICE OF REGIONAL ANESTHESIA

The first report on the use of ultrasound as an aid to nerve location appeared in the anesthesiology literature in 1978.[25] Since the mid 1990s, such reports have become more common as the standard of equipment has improved, costs have decreased, and more portable equipment has become available. Ultrasound has been used as an aid in the performance of blocks of the celiac plexus, psoas compartment, stellate ganglion, and others. However, it is in brachial plexus anesthesia that interest has concentrated.

Fundamentals of ultrasonography

Sound waves above a frequency of 20 000 Hz are ultrasound. An ultrasound device can convert electrical current into sound waves and sound waves into electrical current. It thus acts as both transmitter and receiver. The velocity of transmission of sound waves in a medium depends on the acoustic impedance of that medium, which in turn depends on the density of the medium. When sound waves reach two materials of different acoustic impedance, they are reflected back to different degrees. The greater the impedance, the greater the reflectivity of this signal and the brighter the image seen on the screen. In contrast, fluids transmit sound perfectly and so generate no echoes.[26]

If the emitting source moves away from the receiver, the detected frequency of the wave decreases, and similarly increases as the source moves toward the receiver. This is known as the Doppler effect. In practice, the Doppler effect is used to measure the velocity of blood within a vessel. In order to identify complex structures such as the brachial plexus, high-resolution devices are required with performance in the 7.5–10 MHz range. Availability of the Doppler effect will permit the identification of vascular structures, which may further aid in the location of nerve fibers.

Clinical application

To interpret the images obtained with ultrasound devices, it is necessary in the first instance to have a thorough knowledge not only of the topographic anatomy of the area of interest but also of the cross-sectional anatomy. Ultrasound permits one to non-invasively explore three-dimensional spaces, but only two

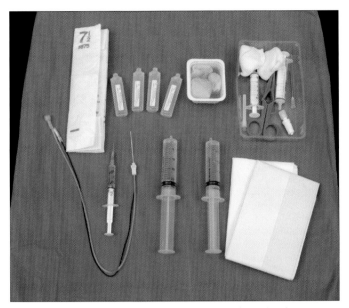

Figure 6.5 Materials required for the performance of peripheral nerve block.

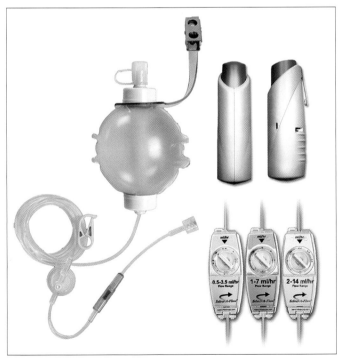

Figure 6.6 Device for continuous plexus block featuring auto delivery large volume patient-controlled analgesia and flow-rate selection.

of these dimensions are visible at any one time. A period of training is therefore necessary to appreciate the benefits of this technology.

In regional anesthesia, ultrasound has been variously used to identify and mark the skin over blood vessels, to guide the needle or catheter to the nerve, to avoid vital structures, to visualize the spread of local anesthetics, and to validate currently used landmarks.[27]

Despite confirmation of correct needle and catheter position with ultrasound, a 100% clinical success rate is not guaranteed. Nevertheless, the reported success rates are similar to those with other techniques.[25] Furthermore, the loss of resolution at greater depths renders the technology less accurate for blocks such as that of the psoas compartment. Devices with the lower frequency of 3.5–5 MHz are required to penetrate these depths.

The value of this technology has been demonstrated in avoiding pneumothorax in infraclavicular blocks by allowing one to visualize the position of the needle tip in relation to vital structures.[28,29] It has led to recommendations for the modification of some approaches depending on patient size, obesity, and sex.[30] It may permit the use of smaller anesthetic volumes and result in a higher success rate and the speedier performance of some blocks.[31]

As the quality and miniaturization of this equipment has improved, it is beginning to move into mainstream clinical practice. A device that aids in peripheral arterial and central venous cannulation and that can be used in regional anesthesia is likely to assume a prominent place in every anesthetic induction room. It may prove particularly valuable in the performance of blocks with potentially serious complications (such as brachial plexus block), improve the success rate and safety profile of regional anesthesia, and act as a teaching and training aid.

References

1. Stoffel A. Eine neue Operation für spastische Lähmungen. Münch Med Woch 1911; 47: 2493–2498.
2. Perthes G. Ueber Leitunganästhesie unter zuhilfenahme elektrischer reizung. Münch Med Woch 1912; 47: 2545–2548.
3. Benhamou D. Axillary plexus block using multiple nerve stimulation: a European view. Reg Anesth Pain Med 2001; 26: 495–498.
4. Montgomery SJ, Raj PP, Nettles D, et al. The use of the nerve stimulator with standard unsheathed needles in nerve blockade. Anesth Analg 1973; 52: 827–831.
5. Raj PP. Ancillary measures to ensure success. Reg Anesth 1980; 5: 9–12.
6. Gold SJ, Duthie DJR. Nerve stimulator current and regional nerve block efficacy. Br J Anaesth 2001; 86: 321.
7. Riegler FX. Brachial plexus block with the nerve stimulator: motor response characteristics at three sites. Reg Anesth 1992; 176: 295–299.
8. Urmey WF, Stanton J, O'Brien S, et al. Inability to consistently elicit a motor response following sensory paresthesia during interscalene block administration. Reg Anesth 1998; 23: 7–57.

9. Auroy Y, Benhamou D, Bargues L, et al. Major complications of regional anesthesia in France. The SOS regional anesthesia hotline service. Anesthesiology 2002; 97: 1274–1279.

10. Plevak D, Linstromberg J, Danielsson D. Paresthesia vs non-paresthesia—the axillary block. Anesthesiology 1983; 59: A216.

11. Selander D, Edshage S, Wolff T. Parasthesiae or no parasthesiae? Nerve lesions after axillary blocks. Acta Anaesth Scand 1979; 23: 27–33.

12. Pither C, Prithvi R, Ford D. The use of peripheral nerve stimulators for regional anesthesia. A review of experimental characteristics, technique and clinical applications. Reg Anesth 1985; 10: 49–58.

13. Shaefer J. Elektrophysiologie I. Wein: Franz Deufficke; 1940.

14. Casey K. Which elements are excited in electrical stimulation of mammalian central nervous system: a review. Brain Res 1975; 98: 417–440.

15. Koslow M, Bak A, Li C. C fibre excitability in the cat. Exp Neurol 1973; 41: 745–753.

16. BeMent SL, Ranck JB. A quantitative study of electrical stimulation of central myelinated fibers. Expo Neurol 1969; 24: 147–170.

17. Ford D, Pither C, Raj P. Electrical characteristics of peripheral nerve stimulators: implications for nerve localization. Reg Anesth 1984; 9: 73–77.

18. Galindo A. Electrical localization of peripheral nerves: instrumentation and clinical experience. Reg Anesth 1983; 8: 49–50.

19. De Andres J, Sala-Blanch X. Peripheral nerve stimulation in the practice of brachial plexus anesthesia: a review. Reg Anesth Pain Med 2001; 26: 478–483.

20. Bashein G, Haschke RH, Ready LB. Electrical nerve location: numerical and electrophoretic comparison of insulated vs uninsulated needles. Anesth Analg 1984; 63: 919–924.

21. [Anonymous]. Technical aspects of peripheral electrical nerve stimulation. Available: http://www.bbraunusa.com/stimuplex/pens1.html.

22. Ansboro F. Method of continuous brachial plexus block. Am J Surg 1946; 71: 716–722.

23. Gale DW, Ramamurthy S, Valley MA. Commonly used neurolytic solutions significantly degrade nylon but not Teflon epidural catheters. Reg Anesth 1996; 21: S51.

24. Copeland SJ, Laxton MA. A new stimulating catheter for continuous peripheral nerve blocks. Reg Anesth Pain Med 2001; 26: 589–590.

25. La Grange P, Foster P, Pretorius L. Application of the Doppler ultrasound blood flow detector in supraclavicular brachial plexus block. Br J Anaesth 1978; 50: 965–967.

26. De Andres J, Sala-Blanch X. Ultrasound in the practice of brachial plexus anesthesia. Reg Anesth Pain Med 2002; 27: 77–89.

27. Peterson MK, Millar FA, Sheppard DG. Ultrasound-guided nerve blocks [editorial]. Br J Anaesth 2002; 88: 621–624.

28. Kapral S, Krafft P, Eisenberger K, et al. Ultrasound-guided supraclavicular approach for regional anesthesia of the brachial plexus. Anesth Analg 1994; 78: 507–513.

29. Ootaki C, Hyashi H, Amano M. Ultrasound-guided infraclavicular brachial plexus block: an alternative technique to anatomical landmark-guided approaches. Reg Anesth Pain Med 2000; 25: 600–604.

30. Greher M, Retzl G, Niel P, et al. Ultrasonographic assessment of topographic anatomy in volunteers suggests a modification of the infraclavicular vertical plexus block. Br J Anaesth 2002; 88: 632–636.

31. Marhofer P, Schrogendorfer K, Koinig H, et al. Ultrasonographic guidance improves sensory block and onset time of three-in-one blocks. Anesth Analg 1997; 85: 854–857.

Part 2

Peripheral nerve blocks

CHAPTER 7

Cervical plexus block

⟐ Indications

Surgical—Superficial neck procedures; excision of thyroglossal and branchial cysts; excision of neck lymph nodes; thyroid and parathyroid surgery; carotid endarterectomy; central venous cannulation; shoulder surgery in combination with inter-scalene block.

Therapeutic—Complex regional pain syndrome; postherpetic neuralgia; postoperative pain.

⟐ Contraindications

Absolute
See Chapter 4.

Relative
Hemorrhagic diathesis; anticoagulation treatment; local neural injury; respiratory compromise; and anatomic distortion (due to previous surgery or trauma).

⟐ Anatomy

The cervical plexus is formed from the ventral rami of the upper four cervical nerves. The dorsal and ventral roots combine to form spinal nerves as they exit through the inter-vertebral foramina. The cervical nerves exit from the cervical spine through gutters in the transverse processes that run in an anterolateral direction, immediately posterior to the vertebral artery. The cervical plexus lies behind the sternocleidomastoid muscle, giving off both superficial (superficial cervical plexus) and deep (deep cervical plexus) branches.

The branches of the *superficial cervical plexus* supply the skin and superficial structures of the head, neck, and shoulder. There are four cutaneous branches, which become sub-cutaneous at the posterior border of the sternocleidomastoid muscle (Fig. 7.1). The lesser occipital and great auricular are derived from the C2 and C3 roots and run in a cephalad direction. The lesser occipital nerve supplies sensation to the upper side of the neck, the upper part of the auricle, and the adjoining skin of the scalp. The great auricular nerve is the largest cutaneous branch and divides into an anterior and a posterior branch. The posterior branch supplies the skin lying behind the ear and the medial and lateral surfaces of the lower part of the auricle. The anterior branch supplies the skin in the lower posterior part of the face and the concave surface of the auricle. The transverse cervical nerve, also from C2 and C3 roots, runs horizontally across the neck and provides sensory innervation to the anterolateral aspect of the neck from the mandible to the sternum. The supraclavicular branch, from the C3 and C4 roots, runs caudally over the clavicle and divides into three branches: medial, intermediate, and lateral. It provides sensory innervation to the lower aspect of the neck, acromial region of the neck, and as far as the second inter-costal space on the chest.

The *deep branches of the cervical plexus* innervate the deeper structures of the neck, including the muscles of the anterior neck and the diaphragm (phrenic nerve).

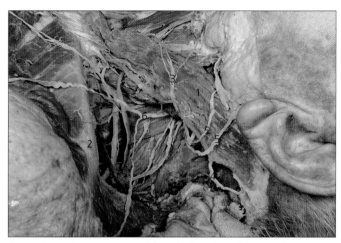

Figure 7.1 Cadaver structures illustrating branches of the superficial cervical plexus. 1, Sternocleidomastoid muscle; 2, clavicle; 3, transverse cervical nerve; 4, lesser occipital nerve; 5, great auricular nerve (anterior and posterior branches); 6, supraclavicular branches (medial, intermediate, and lateral branches).

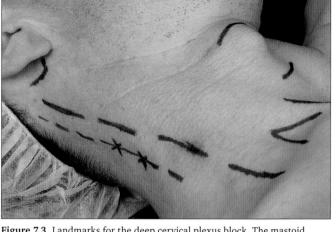

Figure 7.3 Landmarks for the deep cervical plexus block. The mastoid process, suprasternal notch, and transverse process of C6 are identified and marked. A line is drawn along the posterior border of the sternocleidomastoid muscle. A second line is drawn 1 cm posterior to the first line. The C4 transverse process is identified in relation to the transverse process of C6 or at the level of the superior aspect of the thyroid cartilage. Transverse processes of C3 and C2 are located 1.5 and 3 cm proximal from C4.

◈ Surface anatomy

The main landmarks for the superficial cervical plexus block (Fig. 7.2) include mastoid process, suprasternal notch, and posterior border of the sternocleidomastoid muscle at the level of the cricoid cartilage. The sternocleidomastoid muscle and its posterior border can be accentuated by asking the patient to perform a head lift. The external jugular vein crosses the posterior border of the sternocleidomastoid muscle close to the injection site. It can be accentuated by asking the patient to perform a Valsalva maneuver. The carotid artery can be palpated medial to the sternocleidomastoid muscle and indicates the vascular nature of the territory.

The main landmarks for the deep cervical plexus block (Fig. 7.3) include mastoid process; posterior border of the sternocleidomastoid muscle at the level of the cricoid cartilage; C6 transverse process (the most prominent cervical transverse process); and the thyroid cartilage.

◈ Technique

Superficial cervical plexus

As for all regional anesthetic procedures, after checking that emergency equipment is complete and in working order, intravenous access, ECG, pulse oximetry, and blood pressure monitoring are established. Asepsis is observed.

The patient is placed in the supine position with the head facing away from the side to be blocked. The mastoid process and suprasternal notch are identified and marked. The next step is to identify the posterior border of the sternocleidomastoid muscle between these two landmarks. The needle insertion site is marked at the midpoint of the posterior border of the sternocleidomastoid adjacent to the cricoid cartilage (Fig. 7.2).

The needle insertion site is infiltrated with local anesthetic using a 25-G needle. A 23-G needle is then inserted in a perpendicular fashion just behind the posterior border of the sternocleidomastoid muscle (Fig. 7.4). A 'pop' is often felt as the cervical fascia is penetrated. Incremental injection of local

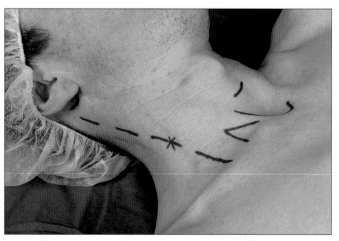

Figure 7.2 Landmarks for the superficial cervical plexus block. The mastoid and suprasternal notch are marked with a pen and the posterior border of the sternocleidomastoid is outlined. The needle insertion point is at the midpoint of this line, which corresponds to the level of the cricoid cartilage.

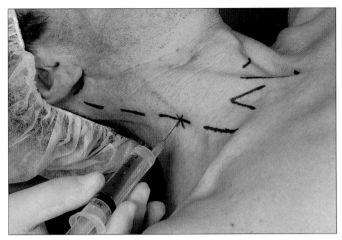

Figure 7.4 Superficial cervical plexus block technique. The needle is first inserted in a perpendicular plane to the skin and behind the posterior border of the sternocleidomastoid muscle. A loss of resistance is felt as the fascia surrounding the sternocleidomastoid is penetrated. Also, subcutaneous injections are made superiorly and inferiorly along the border of the sternocleidomastoid from this point.

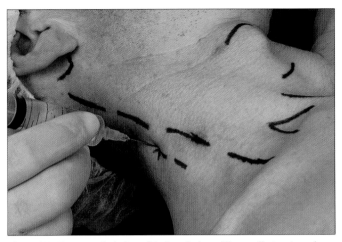

Figure 7.5 Deep cervical plexus block technique. The needle is oriented perpendicular to the skin and slightly caudad until bony contact at 1–2 cm. The needle is withdrawn 1–2 mm and 3–5 mL of local anesthetic is injected.

anesthetic (5 mL) is made with repeated aspiration. This is the preferred block site due to the tight arrangement of the plexus here. Local anesthetic injection should form a contour corresponding to the sternocleidomastoid muscle. The needle is then redirected both superiorly and inferiorly along the posterior border of the sternocleidomastoid while making subcutaneous injections (5-mL injections are made in each direction).

Deep cervical plexus

The mastoid process and transverse process of C6 are identified and marked with a pen (Fig. 7.3). A line is drawn connecting these two points. A second line is drawn parallel and 1 cm posterior to the first line (Fig. 7.3). The transverse process of the fourth cervical vertebrae can be located having previously located the transverse process of the sixth cervical vertebrae in relation to the cricoid cartilage. The transverse process of the fourth cervical vertebrae can also be located by drawing a horizontal line from the superior aspect of the thyroid cartilage. Although a single-injection technique at C4 can be used, block at C3 is also possible. C3 can be located 1.5 cm cephalad from C4.

Needle (23 G) orientation is perpendicular to the skin and slightly caudad (Fig. 7.5) until bony contact at 1–2 cm from the skin. A paresthesia in the distribution of the cervical plexus may be found. At this point the needle is gently withdrawn 1 mm and incremental injections of local anesthetic (3–5 mL) are made with repeated aspiration. The fingers of the palpating hand should be used to fix the skin at the transverse process of the level to be blocked. This decreases the depth of the needle insertion and makes the block both easier and safer to perform.

Adverse effects

Hematoma formation due to puncture of the external jugular vein.

Phrenic nerve block due to its location on the anterior scalene muscle; also *hoarseness*, *dysphagia*, and a *Horners syndrome* due to block of the recurrent laryngeal nerve and the sympathetic chain. Partial block of the brachial plexus is possible, resulting in *upper limb anesthesia*.

Neural injuries are extremely rare. Injury to neuroaxial structures due to proximity is possible; using the needle orientation described decreases this risk.

Local anesthetic toxicity due to injection into the external or internal jugular veins or vertebral artery leads rapidly to toxic reactions.

Clinical Pearls

• Light premedication with midazolam or fentanyl facilitates block placement and significantly decreases patient discomfort during block performance.

• Superficial cervical plexus block is thought to be as effective as the deep cervical plexus block when used for carotid endarterectomy.

• A number of vascular structures are close to this location, so careful and repeated aspirations should be made to avoid accidental intravascular injection of local anesthetic.

Suggested reading

Merle JC, Mazoit JX, Desgranges P, et al. A comparison of two techniques for cervical plexus blockade: evaluation of efficacy and systemic toxicity. Anesth Analg 1999; 89: 1366–1370.

Stoneham MD, Knighton JD. Regional anaesthesia for carotid endarterectomy. Br J Anaesth 1999; 82: 910–919.

CHAPTER 8
Orbital blocks

John McAdoo

Indications

Surgical—Cataract extraction; trabeculectomy; vitrectomy; cryotherapy; panphotocoagulation.
Therapeutic—Postoperative pain relief.

Contraindications

Absolute
See Chapter 4.
Relative
Myopia; anatomic or pathologic abnormalities, which may pose surgical difficulties; raised intraocular pressure; and previous scleral buckling procedures.

Anatomy

Orbital cavity

The superior orbital margin is formed by the frontal bone and contains the supraorbital foramen or notch, through which the superior orbital nerve emerges (Fig. 8.1). The inferior orbital margin is formed laterally by the zygomatic bone and medially by the maxilla. The roof of the orbit is formed by the frontal bone, the lateral or temporal wall by the zygomatic bone. The posterior wall of the orbit consists of the greater and lesser wings of the sphenoid bone. The orbital floor is formed by the

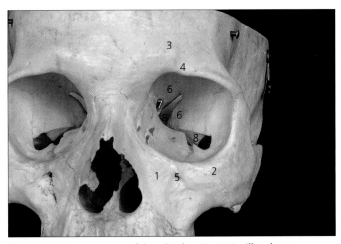

Figure 8.1 Bony structures of the orbital cavity. 1, Maxillary bone; 2, zygomatic bone; 3, frontal bone; 4, supraorbital notch; 5, infraorbital foramen; 6, lesser and greater wings of sphenoid bone; 7, optic canal; 8, superior and inferior orbital fissures.

maxilla, and the medial (nasal) wall of the orbit by the lacrimal bone and the orbital lamina of the ethmoid bone. The superior orbital fissure lies between the greater and lesser wings of the sphenoid bones, and the inferior orbital fissure lies between the maxilla and the superior wing of the sphenoid.

The medial walls of each orbit are parallel to each other (Fig. 8.2). The lateral or temporal wall of each orbit forms an angle of 90° to the contralateral lateral wall. The medial and lateral walls of the orbit make a 45° angle to each other. The

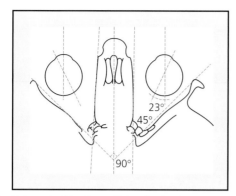

Figure 8.2 Globe and orbit. The medial walls of each orbit are parallel to each other. The lateral (temporal) walls of the orbits form an angle of 90° to each other. The medial and lateral walls of the orbit make a 45° angle with each other.

floor of the orbit inclines at an angle of 10° anteriorly to posteriorly.

The A–P length of the orbit is 40–45 mm (Fig. 8.3) and the orbital volume is approximately 30 mL. The A–P diameter of a normal globe is 24 mm and the horizontal diameter is 23.5 mm. The globe lies eccentrically in the orbit, being displaced medially and superiorly.

Motor nerve supply

The motor nerve supply to the eye (Fig. 8.4) and surrounding structures comes from cranial nerves. The third, fourth, and sixth cranial nerves supply the motor innervation to the recti muscles and partial motor innervation to the levator palpebrae superioris muscle. The seventh cranial nerve supplies motor function to the orbicularis oculi muscles. The parasympathetic nervous system supplies the circular muscle of the iris, while the sympathetic nervous system supplies the radial muscles of the iris and partial innervation to the levator palpebrae superioris muscle. The third, fourth, and sixth cranial nerves enter the orbit via the superior orbital fissure. The third cranial nerve (oculomotor) supplies all recti muscles with the exception of the lateral rectus muscle. The superior oblique muscle is supplied by the fourth cranial nerve (trochlear) and the lateral rectus muscle is supplied by the sixth cranial nerve (abducent). With the exception of the trochlear nerve, the motor nerves lie within the muscle cone formed by the four recti muscles. The nerves enter the muscle cone surrounding the optic nerve via the tendinous ring (annulus of Zinn).

Sensory nerve supply

Sensory supply to the eye (Figs 8.4A, 8.5) and surrounding tissues is via the ophthalmic nerve, which is the first division of the trigeminal nerve. It supplies sensation to the eye, lacrimal gland, conjunctiva, part of the mucous membrane of the nose,

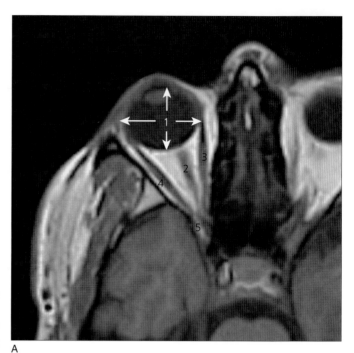

A

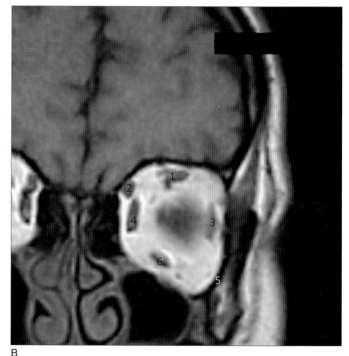

B

Figure 8.3 An MR image of globe and orbit. The A–P length of the orbit is 40–45 mm. The horizontal diameter of a normal globe is 23.5 mm and the A–P diameter is 24 mm. The globe lies eccentrically in the orbit, being displaced medially and superiorly. View **A**: 1, horizontal and AP diameters of eye; 2, optic nerve; 3, medial rectus muscle; 4, lateral rectus muscle; 5, optic canal and nerve. View **B**: 1, superior rectus muscle and levator palpebrae superioris muscles; 2, superior oblique muscle; 3, lateral rectus muscle; 4, medial rectus muscle; 5, orbital margin (J-shaped); 6, interior rectus muscle.

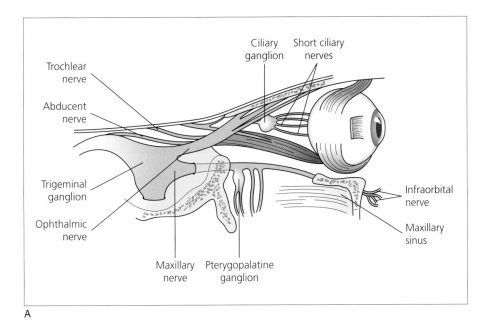

Figure 8.4 Motor supply to the orbit. Lateral (**A**) and frontal (**B**) views.

skin of the nose, eyelids, forehead, and scalp. The ophthalmic nerve enters the orbit via the superior orbital fissure. It is the smallest division of the trigeminal nerve and arises from the anteromedial part of the trigeminal ganglion. Just before entering the superior orbital fissure it divides into three branches: the lacrimal, frontal, and nasociliary nerves.

The *lacrimal nerve* is the smallest branch of the ophthalmic nerve. It enters the orbit via the superior orbital fissure and runs along the upper border of the lateral rectus muscle. It enters the lacrimal gland and gives branches to the lacrimal gland and conjunctiva. Finally it pierces the orbital septum and ends in the skin of the upper eyelid.

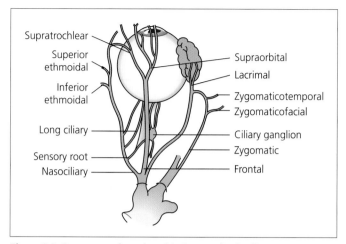

Figure 8.5 Sensory supply to the orbit. See text for details.

The *frontal nerve* is the largest of the branches of the ophthalmic nerve. It enters the orbit via the superior orbital fissure outside the muscle cone. It runs superiorly to the levator palpebrae superioris. It divides into the supraorbital and supratrochlear nerves. The supraorbital nerve passes through the supraorbital foramen or notch and gives branches to the conjunctiva and eyelid. It then continues and supplies the skin of the scalp almost to the lambdoid suture. The supratrochlear nerve emerges from the orbit between the trochlea and the supraorbital foramen. It supplies sensation to the conjunctiva and skin of the upper eyelid and the skin of the lower forehead.

The *nasociliary nerve* enters the orbit via the superior orbital fissure within the tendinous ring close to the oculomotor nerve and ophthalmic artery. It gives off the long posterior ciliary nerves and branches to the ciliary ganglion. It also gives off the anterior and posterior ethmoid nerves.

Optic nerve

The optic nerve enters the orbit via the optic canal. It enters the muscle cone via the tendinous ring surrounded by dura mater. It contains the central retinal artery and vein. The ophthalmic artery lies lateral to the optic nerve initially, and then crosses superiorly to lie medial to the optic nerve within the muscle cone. The ophthalmic venous plexus also lies in close proximity.

Arterial supply

The ophthalmic artery is a branch of the internal carotid artery as it emerges from the cavernous sinus. It enters the orbital cavity through the optic canal below and lateral to the optic nerve. It enters the muscle cone via the tendinous ring and runs lateral to the optic nerve and medial to the oculomotor and abducent nerves, ciliary ganglion, and lateral rectus muscle. It crosses above the optic nerve to reach the medial wall of the muscle cone and runs anterior between the superior oblique and the medial rectus muscles. It divides into two branches: the supratrochlear and dorsal nasal. Other branches are the central retinal artery, lacrimal artery, and the long and short posterior ciliary arteries. Branches also supply the muscles, eyelids, and meninges.

Venous drainage

Venous drainage of the orbit is via the ophthalmic veins, of which there are two. The superior ophthalmic vein runs with the ophthalmic artery and has corresponding tributaries. It passes through the superior fissure and ends in the cavernous sinus. The inferior orbital vein begins in a venous complex on the floor and medial wall of the orbit. It may join the superior ophthalmic vein or may empty directly into the cavernous sinus via the inferior orbital sinus. The central retinal vein traverses the optic nerve to end in either the superior ophthalmic vein or the cavernous sinus.

Ocular muscles

The muscles of the eyelids (Fig. 8.4B) include the levator palpebrae superioris and the orbicularis oculi muscles. The orbital muscles are the four recti muscles and the superior and inferior oblique muscles. The recti muscles arise from the semitendinous ring, which surrounds the optic canal. The muscles penetrate the fascial sheath of the eyeball (Tenon's capsule) and are inserted in the sclera 5–6 mm posterior to the corneoscleral junction. The superior oblique muscle arises from the body of the sphenoid and, having traversed the trochlea, passes backward and is inserted into the sclera posterior to the equator. The inferior oblique muscle arises from the orbital surface of the maxilla medially and is inserted into the lateral part of the sclera behind the equator.

Tenon's capsule (fascial sheath of the eyeball)

Tenon's capsule (Fig. 8.6) is a thin membrane that envelops the eyeball from the optic nerve to the corneoscleral junction. It separates the eye from the orbital fat and forms a capsule within which the eye moves. It is separated from the sclera by the episcleral space. Tenon's capsule is penetrated posteriorly by the ciliary vessels and nerves and fuses with the sheath of the optic nerve. Anteriorly, it fuses with the sclera just behind the corneoscleral junction. The tendons of the recti muscles penetrate the capsule anteriorly.

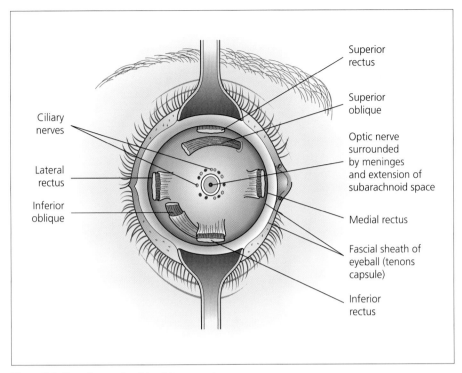

Figure 8.6 Tenon's capsule with orbit removed.

Labels in figure:
Ciliary nerves
Lateral rectus
Inferior oblique
Superior rectus
Superior oblique
Optic nerve surrounded by meninges and extension of subarachnoid space
Medial rectus
Fascial sheath of eyeball (tenons capsule)
Inferior rectus

◈ Surface anatomy

Extraconal retrobulbar and lateral peribulbar blocks

The needle insertion points for the extraconal retrobular (Fig. 8.7) and lateral peribulbar blocks is at the lowest margin of the inferior rim of the orbit. This approximates to the junction of the medial two-thirds and the lateral one-third of the lower lid. This will give the greatest distance from the globe and avoids the inferior rectus muscle.

Medial peribulbar block

The plica semilunaris, which lies temporal to the caruncle, is the landmark for the medial peribulbar block (Fig. 8.8).

Sub-Tenon block

The point of insertion for the sub-Tenon block (Fig. 8.9) is the point on the conjunctiva halfway between the inferior and medial recti muscles 4 mm from the corneoscleral junction.

◈ Technique

As for all regional anesthetic procedures, after checking that the emergency equipment is complete and in working order, intravenous access, ECG, pulse oximetry, and blood pressure monitoring are established. Asepsis is observed.

Extraconal retrobulbar block

The side to be anesthetized and the axial length of the globe are verified. The axial length dictates which block will be used because an axial length greater than 26 mm is a relative contraindication to retrobulbar block. The patient lies in the supine position.

The operator stands on the side to be blocked, below the patient's shoulder. The local anesthetic cream, which is applied 1 h before surgery to the skin of the lower lid on the side to be anesthetized, is removed in the operating theater when the skin is prepared with antiseptic solution. The inferior orbital margin is identified at the junction of the medial two-thirds and lateral one-third of the lower eyelid. With the eye in the primary or neutral position, the inferior lid is indented, gently displacing the eye upward and medially within the orbit. A 32-mm 27-G Atkinson tipped needle on a 5-mL syringe is inserted between the indenting finger and the inferior orbital margin. The needle is directed initially vertically in the sagittal and coronal planes, using the indenting finger to maintain the direction of the needle. The needle is inserted to a depth of 16 mm, which ensures that the tip of the needle is past the greater diameter of the eye.

The needle is now angled parallel to the orbital floor and the lateral wall of the orbit, and is inserted to its full depth

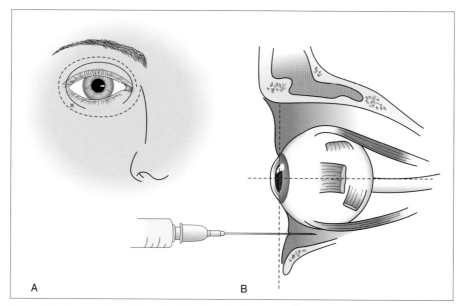

Figure 8.7 Extraconal retrobulbar block. Landmarks (**A**) and needle insertion at the lowest margin of the inferior rim of the orbit (**B**). The needle passes backward in a sagittal plane and parallel to the orbital floor and lateral wall.

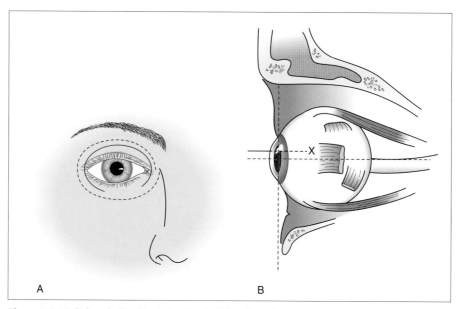

Figure 8.8 Medial peribulbar block. Landmarks (**A**) and needle insertion at the medial side of the caruncle (**B**). The needle passes backward in a sagittal plane and parallel to the medial orbital wall. Depth of insertion can range between 12 mm to a maximal needle insertion of 25 mm, as measured by observing the needle or hub junction reach the plane of the iris, as shown.

or 25 mm for a lateral peribulbar technique. This technique reduces significantly the risk of the needle entering the muscle cone. Following aspiration, 4 mL of lidocaine 2% and 1:200 000 adrenaline (epinephrine) plus 75 IU/mL hyaluronidase (Hyalase®) is injected slowly. The needle is removed and gentle pressure is applied to the closed eye. Assessing lateral and vertical eye movement verifies the efficacy of the block. Finally the eye is assessed for the presence of chemosis and hemorrhage. A Honan balloon is applied to the eye and inflated to 35 mmHg. This reduces the intraocular pressure prior to surgery.

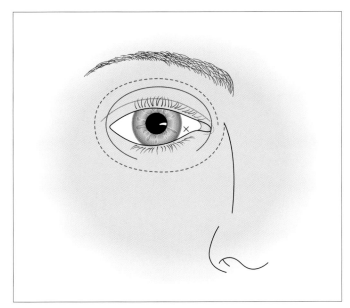

Figure 8.9 Landmarks for sub-Tenon block. The point of needle insertion is halfway between the inferior and medial recti muscles 4 mm from the corneoscleral junction.

Medial peribulbar block

The patient lies in the supine position. The operator stands on the side to be blocked, at the patient's shoulder. With the eye in the primary position, the lids are separated to identify the plica semilunaris medially adjacent to the caruncle. Local anesthetic drops are applied topically to the conjunctiva of the eye. A 32-mm 27-G Atkinson tipped needle on a syringe is angled tangentially to the globe, piercing the conjunctiva at the plica semilunaris. When the tip of the needle touches the medial wall of the orbit, the direction of the needle is changed to the vertical in the sagittal and coronal planes. The needle is inserted until its tip meets the lacrimal crest—usually at a depth of 12 mm. Following aspiration, 2–4 mL of bupivacaine 0.5% is injected. Assessing lateral and vertical eye movement verifies the efficacy of the block. Finally the eye is assessed for the presence of chemosis and hemorrhage.

Sub-Tenon block

The patient lies in the supine position. The operator stands on the side to be blocked, at the patient's shoulder. Local anesthetic drops are applied topically to the conjunctiva of the eye. Antiseptic drops are also applied. An appropriate left- or right-eye speculum is carefully placed, separating the eyelids.

The conjunctiva midway between the medial and inferior recti muscles is gently picked up with Moorfield forceps 3–4 mm from the limbus. Blunt-tipped curved Westcott spring scissors, with the tips pointing away from the globe, are used to open the conjunctiva. The conjunctiva and Tenon capsule

are separated from the sclera with the tips of the scissors. A curved blunt 19-G sub-Tenon cannula is inserted gently under the conjunctiva, following the curve of the globe until a slight resistance is felt. Then 4 mL of lidocaine 2% with 1:200 000 adrenaline is injected beneath the Tenon capsule. A slight resistance to the injection should be felt but resistance should not be excessive. The onset of complete block will take approximately 15 min. Assessing lateral and vertical eye movement verifies the efficacy of the block. The eye is assessed for the presence of chemosis and hemorrhage.

Adverse effects

Globe perforation has been reported with all techniques described. At particular risk are myopic eyes with an axial length greater than 26 mm and eyes that have undergone scleral buckling operations. This is due to a thin sclera, staphylomas, and the increased diameters of the eye. This is a serious sight-threatening complication.

Central spread of local anesthetic to the brain, leading to cardiovascular system instability and respiratory depression, may occur. This is a life-threatening complication.

Retrobulbar hemorrhage may be due to arterial or venous hemorrhage and is potentially sight-threatening.

Optic nerve trauma is a very rare, sight-threatening complication.

Central retinal artery or vein occlusion is associated with patients with atherosclerotic vascular disease. Avoid local anesthetics containing adrenaline.

Ocular muscle dysfunction may be transient or permanent. This complication is attributed to either direct myotoxicity of local anesthetic agents or hemorrhage into muscles due to trauma.

Subconjunctival chemosis and *subconjunctival hemorrhage*, which resolve spontaneously.

Clinical Pearls

• Check axial length before any orbital local anesthetic procedure. If measurement is not available (e.g. for a patient undergoing a trabeculectomy) ask the patient about wearing corrective lenses or glasses for distance vision.

• Always ask patients to maintain their eye in the primary or neutral position during local anesthetic procedures.

• For cataract extraction, absolute eye akinesia is not necessary.

Subcutaneous hemorrhage at site of transcutaneous injections; this resolves spontaneously.

Corneal abrasion due to trauma of speculum insertion may decrease operative view for the surgeon.

Suggested reading

Fichman RA, Hoffman J. Anaesthesia for cataract surgery and its complications. Curr Opin Ophthalmol 1994; 5: 21–27.

Wong DHW. Regional anaesthesia for intraocular surgery. Can J Anaesth 1993: 40; 635–657.

CHAPTER 9
Brachial plexus anatomy

Before selection of technique, it is important to have a thorough understanding of brachial plexus anatomy. The plexus is composed of roots, trunks, divisions, cords, and branches (Fig. 9.1). The brachial plexus stems from the ventral rami of the C5 to T1 nerve roots in the majority of individuals. Approximately 15% of patients may have contributions to the brachial plexus from the C4 or T2 nerve roots creating a 'prefixed' or 'postfixed' plexus (see Fig. 10.7). The cervical roots emerge from the intervertebral foramina and lie on a sulcus on the vertebral transverse processes between the anterior and posterior tubercles to which the scalene muscles are attached. Immediately lateral to the transverse processes of the cervical vertebrae, the nerve roots are sheathed in the prevertebral fascia. The nerve roots then travel between the scalene muscles and form three trunks (upper, middle, and lower). The interscalene groove is a palpable surface anatomy depression between the anterior and middle scalene muscles; it allows clinicians easy and reliable access to the roots and

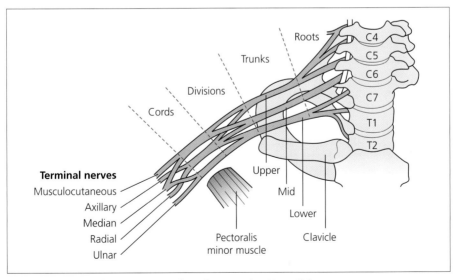

Figure 9.1 Brachial plexus anatomy. L, lateral; P, posterior; M, medial.

trunks of the plexus. The roots are posterior to the vertebral artery—an important anatomic relation for the interscalene block.

The dorsal scapular nerve (to rhomboids) and the long thoracic nerve (to serratus anterior) arise from the C5 and C5, 6, and 7 roots, respectively. The upper (C5, 6) and lower (C8, T1) pairs of roots merge to form the upper and lower trunks of the brachial plexus, while the middle root (C7) continues as the middle trunk. The lower trunk is smaller than the others, and is frequently derived entirely from the eighth cervical nerve. The nerve to subclavius arises from the roots of C5 and C6 where they join to form the upper trunk, which also gives off the suprascapular nerve (to supra- and infraspinatus muscles and the shoulder joint). The trunks are formed in the lower part of the posterior triangle of the neck, between the sternocleidomastoid and trapezius muscles and above the middle third of the clavicle. The trunks travel to the margin of the first rib and divide into anterior and posterior divisions.

RELATIONS

In the neck, the brachial plexus lies in the posterior triangle, being covered by the skin, platysma, and deep fascia; it is crossed by the supraclavicular nerves, the inferior belly of the omohyoid, the external jugular vein, and the transverse cervical artery. It emerges between the anterior and medial scalene muscles; its upper part lies above the third part of the subclavian artery, while the trunk formed by the union of the eighth cervical and first thoracic is placed behind the artery. The plexus next passes behind the clavicle.

Each trunk divides into an anterior and a posterior division behind the clavicle. Divisions then form three cords as they pass under the clavicle and around the humeral head, where they are joined by the axillary artery. The cords are labeled as the lateral, medial, and posterior cords; they are named as such based on the relative anatomic position to the axillary artery. At the outer border of the first rib, the upper two anterior divisions unite to form the lateral cord, the anterior division of the lower trunk runs on as the medial cord, while all three posterior divisions unite to form the posterior cord. The lateral and medial cords provide ventral innervation to the upper limb, with the posterior cord providing dorsal innervation. The cords enter the axilla from above the axillary artery and lie lateral, medial, and posterior to the middle part of the artery, behind the pectoralis minor muscle. The cords divide at the border of the pectoralis minor muscle into five major peripheral nerves, which provide innervation to the upper extremity. The five nerves of the brachial plexus are the axillary, musculocutaneous, radial, median, and ulnar nerves.

The cords and the artery are surrounded by a thin fascial sheath called the axillary sheath. The sheath is a collection of connective tissue surrounding the neurovascular structures of the brachial plexus. It is a continuum of the prevertebral fascia, which invests the scalene muscles in the neck. The sheath is a multicompartmental structure formed by thin layers of fibrous tissue surrounding the plexus in thin membranes and extending inward to create discrete fascial septae. Nerves are thus enmeshed in this tissue rather than lying separate and distinct. These compartments may limit the circumferential spread of injected solutions, thereby requiring separate injections into each compartment for maximal nerve block. However, proximal connections between compartments have been identified, which may account for the success of single-injection techniques.

Lateral and medial pectoral nerves from their respective cords supply the pectoralis major and minor. The musculocutaneous nerve from the lateral cord enters coracobrachialis, supplying it and going on to supply biceps and brachialis; it becomes the lateral cutaneous nerve of the forearm at the lateral side of the biceps tendon at the elbow. Lateral and medial roots from their respective cords unite to form the median nerve, which crosses in front of the brachial artery at the middle of the arm and lies medial to the artery at the elbow. The ulnar nerve arises from the medial cord between the axillary artery and vein, and passes down the medial aspect of the arm to lie behind the base of the medial epicondyle at the elbow. The radial nerve from the posterior cord passes posteriorly through an intermuscular space to spiral round the back of the humerus and enter the cubital fossa, where it lies in a deep plane between brachioradialis and brachialis. The radial nerve gives off the posterior cutaneous nerve of the arm in the axilla, and the lower lateral cutaneous nerve of the arm and posterior cutaneous nerve of the forearm at the back of the humerus. The posterior cord also gives off two subscapular nerves (to subscapularis and teres major), the thoracodorsal nerve (to latissimus dorsi), and the axillary (circumflex humeral) nerve; the latter winds round the back of the humerus to supply deltoid and a small area of skin at the upper lateral part of the arm.

BRANCHES OF THE BRACHIAL PLEXUS

The branches of the brachial plexus may be arranged into two groups: those given off above and those below the clavicle.

Supraclavicular branches (from roots or trunks)

- Dorsal scapular C5.
- Suprascapular C5, 6.
- Nerve to subclavius C5, 6.
- Long thoracic C5, 6, 7.
- To longus colli and scaleni C5, 6, 7, 8.

Infraclavicular branches

The infraclavicular branches are derived from the three cords of the brachial plexus.

Lateral cord

- Musculocutaneous C5, 6, 7.
- Lateral pectoral C5, 6, 7.
- Lateral head of median nerve C6, 7.

Medial cord

- Medial pectoral C8, T1.
- Medial cutaneous nerve of forearm C8, T1.
- Medial cutaneous nerve of arm C8, T1.
- Ulnar C8, T1.
- Medial head of median nerve C8, T1.

Posterior cord

- Upper subscapular C5, 6.
- Lower subscapular C5, 6.
- Thoracodorsal C5, 6, 7.
- Axillary C5, 6.
- Radial C6, 7, 8, T1.

The median nerve

The median nerve (C6 to T1) extends along the middle of the arm and forearm to the hand. As it descends through the arm, it lies at first lateral to the brachial artery; about the level of the insertion of the coracobrachialis it crosses the artery—usually in front of, but occasionally behind it—and lies on its medial side at the elbow, where it is situated behind the bicipital fascia and is separated from the elbow joint by brachialis. In the forearm it passes between the two heads of the pronator teres and crosses the ulnar artery, but is separated from this vessel by the deep head of the pronator teres muscle. It descends beneath the flexor digitorum superficialis, and lies on flexor digitorum profundus, to within 5 cm of the wrist flexor retinaculum; here it becomes more superficial and is situated between the tendons of the flexor digitorum superficialis and flexor carpi radialis. Here it lies behind, and rather to the radial side of, the tendon of the palmaris longus, and is covered by the skin and fascia. It then passes behind the wrist flexor retinaculum.

The ulnar nerve

The ulnar nerve (C8 to T1) is smaller than the median nerve and lies at first behind it, but diverges from it in its course down the arm. At its origin it lies medial to the axillary artery, and bears the same relation to the brachial artery as far as the middle of the arm. Here it pierces the medial intermuscular septum, runs obliquely across the medial head of the triceps muscle, and descends to the groove between the medial epicondyle and the olecranon, accompanied by the superior ulnar collateral artery. At the elbow, it rests on the back of the medial epicondyle, and enters the forearm between the two heads of the flexor carpi ulnaris. In the forearm, it descends along the ulnar side lying on the flexor digitorum profundus; its upper half is covered by the flexor carpi ulnaris, its lower half lies on the lateral side of the muscle, fascia, and skin. In the upper third of the forearm, it is separated from the ulnar artery by a considerable interval, but in the rest of its extent lies close to the medial side of the artery. About 5 cm above the wrist it ends by dividing into a dorsal and a ventral branch.

The radial nerve

The radial nerve (C5 to T1), the largest branch of the brachial plexus, is the continuation of the posterior cord of the plexus. It descends behind the first part of the axillary artery and the upper part of the brachial artery, and in front of the tendons of the latissimus dorsi and teres major. It then winds around from the medial to the lateral side of the humerus in a groove between the medial and lateral heads of the triceps. It pierces the lateral intermuscular septum and passes between the brachialis and brachioradialis to the front of the lateral epicondyle, where it divides into a superficial and a deep branch.

The superficial branch of the radial nerve

The superficial branch of the radial nerve passes along the front of the radial side of the forearm to the commencement of its lower third. It lies at first slightly lateral to the radial artery, concealed beneath brachioradialis. In the middle third of the forearm, it lies behind the same muscle, close to the lateral side of the artery. It leaves the artery about 7 cm above the wrist, passes beneath the tendon of brachioradialis, and piercing the deep fascia divides into two branches. The lateral branch, the smaller, supplies the skin of the radial side and ball of the thumb, joining with the ventral branch of the lateral cutaneous nerve of the forearm. The medial branch communicates, above the wrist, with the dorsal branch of the lateral cutaneous nerve of the forearm, and on the back of the hand with the dorsal branch of the ulnar nerve.

The deep branch of the radial nerve

The deep branch of the radial nerve winds to the back of the forearm around the lateral side of the radius between the two planes of fibers of the supinator, and continues downward between the superficial and deep layers of muscles to the middle of the forearm. Diminished in size, it descends as the dorsal interosseous nerve on the interosseous membrane, in front of the extensor pollicis longus, to the back of the wrist,

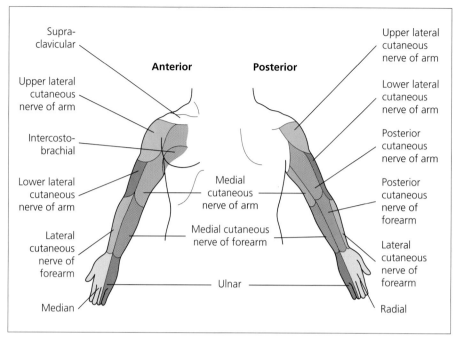

Figure 9.2 Cutaneous innervation of the upper limb.

where it presents a gangliform enlargement from which filaments are distributed to the ligaments and articulations of the wrist.

The sensory (Figs 9.2, 9.3) and motor innervation of the upper limb is clinically important. Knowledge of sensory innervation helps determine which cutaneous nerve distributions within a surgical field require blockade. Motor innervation is clinically relevant as a means of matching a peripheral nerve stimulation response to a particular nerve being stimulated. As the arm has multiple innervation, assessment of block efficacy is best achieved by assessing function unique to each nerve. It is important to remember that significant variation in the structure of the brachial plexus occurs, with seven major configurations described.

The approaches to the brachial plexus include the interscalene, supraclavicular, infraclavicular, axillary, and midhumeral approaches. In relation to the brachial plexus anatomy, the interscalene block is performed at the level of the trunks, whereas the supraclavicular block is performed where the divisions are transitioning into cords. The infraclavicular block is performed at the proximal cord level and the axillary block is performed where the terminal nerves emerge. The midhumeral approach occurs well after the peripheral nerves have been formed.

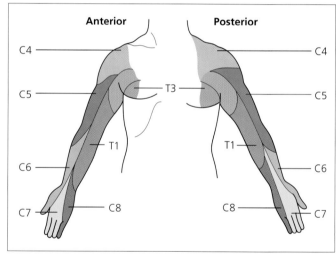

Figure 9.3 Sensory dermatomes of the upper limb.

Suggested reading

Williams PL, Warwick R, Dyson M, et al. Gray's anatomy. 37th edn. London: Churchill Livingstone; 1989.

CHAPTER 10

Interscalene block

Indications

Surgical—Surgical procedures of the clavicle, shoulder, upper arm, and forearm (exception being the medial aspect).

Therapeutic—Shoulder and upper arm pain ('frozen shoulder'); humeroscapular periarthritis; poststroke pain; postherpetic neuralgia; lymphedema after breast surgery; vascular diseases and injuries; complex regional pain syndrome; post-amputation pain; tumor-related pain; pain management for shoulder rehabilitation therapy; prolonged postoperative analgesia (continuous technique).

Contraindications

Absolute
See Chapter 4.

Relative
Hemorrhagic diathesis; anticoagulation treatment; chronic obstructive airways disease; contralateral paresis of the phrenic or recurrent laryngeal nerves; and distorted anatomy (due to previous surgery or trauma).

Anatomy

The cervical nerves exit from the cervical spine through gutters in the transverse processes that run in an anterolateral direction, immediately posterior to the vertebral artery. The cervical nerves enter a facial space in the posterior triangle of the neck between the anterior and middle scalene muscles called the interscalene compartment (Fig. 10.1). The interscalene block is performed at the level of the cricoid cartilage (C6). Important anatomic relations (Fig. 10.2) include the external jugular vein, which crosses the posterior border of the sternocleidomastoid muscle at this point, the phrenic nerve on the anterior scalene muscle, and the vertebral artery.

Surface anatomy

The main landmarks for the interscalene block (Fig. 10.3) include clavicle; sternal notch; cricoid cartilage; sternal and clavicular heads of the sternocleidomastoid muscle—these can be accentuated by asking the patient to perform a head lift; interscalene groove—both scalene muscles descend to the first rib and can be identified by asking the patient to inhale deeply, because they contract before the sternocleidomastoid muscle; and the external jugular vein—which can be accentuated by asking the patient to perform a Valsalva maneuver. A skin marker should routinely be used to delineate the anatomic structures before performing the block.

Technique

As for all regional anesthetic procedures, after checking that emergency equipment is complete and in working order,

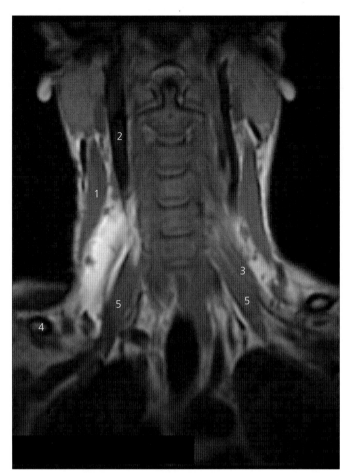

Figure 10.1 Coronal T1-weighted MR image showing the anatomy of the cervical region relevant to interscalene block (post contrast). Note relation of anterior and medial scalene muscles on the side contralateral to the injected contrast. 1, Sternocleidomastoid muscle; 2, common carotid artery; 3, middle scalene muscle; 4, clavicle; 5, anterior scalene muscle.

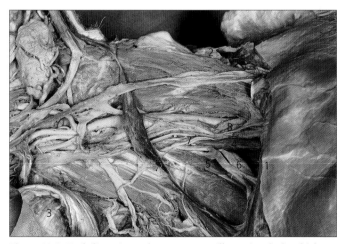

Figure 10.2 Neck dissection cadaver structures illustrating the brachial plexus. 1, Clavicle; 2, cricoid cartilage; 3, retracted sternocleidomastoid muscle; 4, anterior scalene muscle; 5, middle scalene muscle; 6, brachial plexus; 7, phrenic nerve; 8, internal jugular vein.

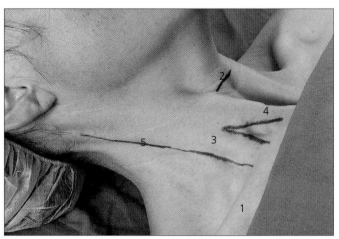

Figure 10.3 Landmarks for the interscalene block. Further accentuation of the anatomy can be achieved by asking patients to lift their head up against resistance (with the head turned to the side). Additionally, when palpating the interscalene groove, the groove can be better appreciated by asking the patient to sniff. 1, Clavicle; 2, cricoid cartilage; 3, sternal head of the sternocleidomastoid muscle; 4, clavicular head of the sternocleidomastoid muscle; 5, posterior border of the sternocleidomastoid muscle.

intravenous access, ECG, pulse oximetry, and blood pressure monitoring are established. Asepsis is observed.

The patient is placed in the supine position with the head facing away from the side to be blocked. The patient is asked to elevate the head slightly to bring the clavicular head of the sternocleidomastoid muscle into prominence. The palpating finger is placed behind the sternocleidomastoid muscle and the patient is instructed to end the head lift (Fig. 10.4). The finger now lies on the belly of the anterior scalene muscle, and with lateral movement of the finger to the lateral edge of this muscle, the groove between the anterior and middle scalene muscles (interscalene groove) is encountered (Fig. 10.5). The injection site in the interscalene groove lies at the level of the

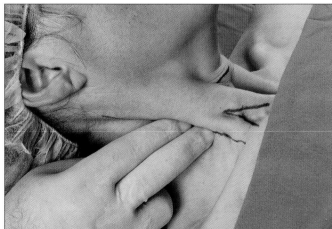

Figure 10.4 Locating the interscalene groove. The palpating fingers are placed deep to the sternocleidomastoid muscle.

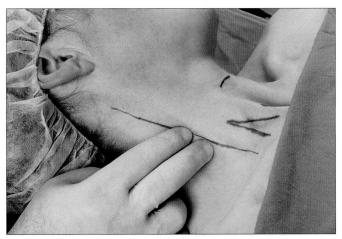

Figure 10.5 Locating the interscalene groove. The fingers are rolled laterally until a groove behind the posterior border of sternocleidomastoid is identified.

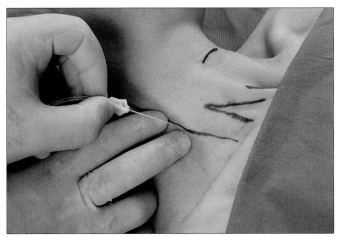

Figure 10.6 Interscalene block technique. The needle is inserted into the interscalene groove at the level of the cricoid cartilage and advanced into the groove with an inward, downward, and backward orientation. The index and middle finger of the palpating hand are placed over the interscalene groove and the skin over the groove is stretched.

cricoid opposite the transverse process of C6 (Chassaignac tubercle).

The needle insertion point is infiltrated with local anesthetic using a 25-G needle. A 35–50-mm 21-G insulated needle is used. The index and middle fingers of the palpating hand should be firmly seated in the interscalene groove. To assure stability of both hands, all fingers not in use should be resting on the neighboring structures. The direction of needle insertion runs inward, slightly dorsally, and 30–40° caudally (backward, inward, and downward) (Fig. 10.6). This needle direction takes into account the orientation of the gutter of the transverse processes of the cervical vertebrae, on which the cervical roots lie. It also acts as a safety technique to decrease the risk of intervertebral needle insertion. The stimulating current is set at 1.0 mA, 2 Hz, and 0.1 ms. The needle is advanced slowly until the appropriate muscle response is obtained: shoulder, elbow, index finger, or thumb movement. The needle position is adjusted while decreasing the current to 0.35 mA with maintenance of the muscle response.

Muscle responses that indicate a less than optimal final needle location include diaphragmatic contraction. The phrenic nerve lies on the anterior scalene muscle and is thus a needle location that is too anterior to the plexus. Muscle contraction of the posterior compartment muscles of the shoulder indicates suprascapular nerve stimulation, a final needle position that is too posterior. Failure to obtain motor response to nerve stimulation should prompt withdrawal of the needle and reinsertion in a 5–10% angle anterior or posterior to the initial insertion plane.

Incremental injections of local anesthetic (40 mL) are made with repeated aspiration. This volume is sufficient for an adequate block of the brachial plexus and the caudal part of the cervical plexus (Fig. 10.7). Digital pressure is applied proximal to injection (Fig. 10.8) to promote distal spread of

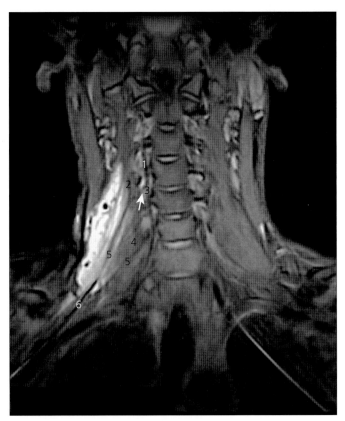

Figure 10.7 Coronal fat-saturated MR image after injection of 30 mL of contrast. Note C4 nerve root joining C5 nerve root, creating a 'prefixed' brachial plexus. Spread of contrast reaches the level of the upper border of C4 and caudad to the level of clavicle. 1, Vertebral artery; 2, C4 root; 3, C5 root; 4, posterior and middle scalene muscles; 5, brachial plexus elements; 6, brachial plexus.

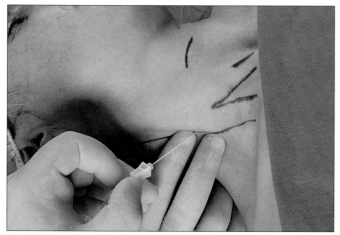

Figure 10.8 Interscalene block technique. Proximal digital pressure promotes distal spread of local anesthetic.

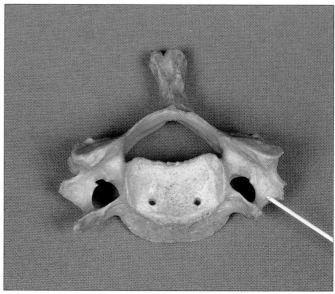

Figure 10.9 The final needle location on the C6 vertebra and the foramen that contains the vertebral artery. The cervical roots are posterior to the vertebral artery.

local anesthetic; this is to facilitate reaching the lower roots of the plexus. The lower roots of the plexus may not be anesthetized due to the proximal injection site with this technique.

Continuous technique

Continuous interscalene block requires modification of the single-shot technique in order to facilitate insertion of the catheter into the brachial plexus sheath. As with other continuous nerve block techniques, the initial dose of local anesthetic is usually injected and only then is the infusion of a more dilute local anesthetic initiated.

Once the local anesthetic is injected, the catheter is carefully inserted some 5 cm beyond the tip of the needle while keeping the needle immobile. When the catheter meets resistance at the tip of the needle, the needle may be repositioned at a different angle or rotated to facilitate advancement of the catheter. Once the catheter is inserted, the needle is withdrawn while simultaneously advancing the catheter to prevent its dislodgment from the brachial plexus sheath.

✧ Adverse effects

Hoarseness due to block of the recurrent laryngeal nerve.

Unilateral paralysis of the diaphragm due to proximity of phrenic nerve on anterior scalene muscle.

Horner syndrome due to stellate ganglion block.

Neural injuries are extremely rare.

Local anesthetic toxicity due to intravascular injection into the vertebral artery or other cervical vessels, leading rapidly to

toxic reactions. The vertebral artery runs in the foramen of the C6 cervical transverse process, not far from final needle location with the interscalene block. This relation can be seen on the C6 cervical vertebra (Fig. 10.9).

Epidural or subarachnoid injection: high epidural block or total spinal block, both requiring immediate treatment. Injection in a caudal direction (avoiding horizontal orientation) with short needles reduces this risk. The distance from skin to the spinal canal can be as short as 0.5 cm.

Pneumothorax is unlikely with correct technique.

Pressure on the carotid artery is rare and transient due to volume of injectate.

Clinical Pearls

• If an upper arm tourniquet is to be used then the interscalene block must be combined with block of the intercostobrachial nerve by subcutaneous injection in the axilla.

• The twitches of the deltoid muscle are sufficient. There does not seem to be any increase in success rate after obtaining more distal twitch responses.

Suggested reading

Borgeat A, Ekatodramis G, Kalberer F, et al. Acute and nonacute complications associated with interscalene block and shoulder surgery: a prospective study. Anesthesiology 2001; 95: 875–880.

Lehtipalo S, Koskinen LO, Johansson G, et al. Continuous interscalene brachial plexus block for postoperative analgesia following shoulder surgery. Acta Anaesthesiol Scand 1999; 43: 258–264.

Long TR, Wass CT, Burkle CM. Perioperative interscalene blockade: an overview of its history and current clinical use. J Clin Anesth 2002; 14: 546–556.

Winnie AP. Interscalene brachial plexus block. Anesth Analg 1970; 49: 455–466.

CHAPTER 11

Supraclavicular block

✧ Indications

Surgical—Surgical procedures of the proximal humerus, elbow, forearm, and hand.
Therapeutic—Complex regional pain syndrome; post-amputation pain; postherpetic neuralgia; tumor-related pain; vascular diseases and injuries; prolonged postoperative analgesia (continuous technique).

✧ Contraindications

Absolute
See Chapter 4.
Relative
Hemorrhagic diathesis; anticoagulation therapy; local neural injury; contralateral paresis of the phrenic or recurrent laryngeal nerves; and contralateral pneumothorax or pneumonectomy.

✧ Anatomy

In the neck the brachial plexus lies in the posterior triangle (Fig. 11.1), covered by the investing layer of deep cervical fascia, platysma, and skin. It is crossed by the supraclavicular nerves, the inferior belly of the omohyoid muscle, the external jugular vein, and the transverse cervical artery and vein. It emerges between the anterior scalene and middle scalene muscles; its upper part lies above the third part of the

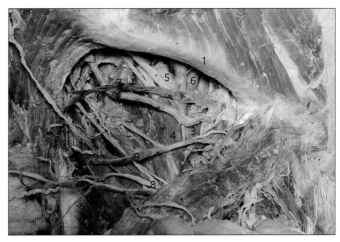

Figure 11.1 Cadaver structures illustrating anatomy pertinent to the supraclavicular subclavian perivascular technique. 1, Clavicle; 2, sternocleidomastoid muscle; 3, anterior scalene muscle; 4, middle scalene muscle; 5, brachial plexus; 6, subclavian artery; 7, transverse cervical artery and vein; 8, branches of cervical plexus; 9, omohyoid muscle retracted upward.

subclavian artery, while the lower trunk formed by the union of the eighth cervical and first thoracic is placed behind the artery; the plexus next passes behind the clavicle.

✧ Surface anatomy

Important landmarks for the supraclavicular block include the interscalene groove behind the posterior border of the

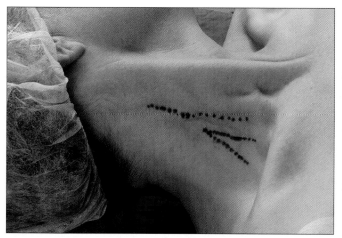

Figure 11.2 Landmarks for the supraclavicular block. The posterior border of the sternocleidomastoid muscle and interscalene groove are identified. The interscalene groove is followed toward the clavicle. The subclavian pulse is palpable above the clavicle in the interscalene groove.

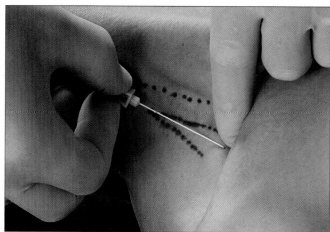

Figure 11.3 Supraclavicular block technique: needle orientation. The needle is first inserted immediately posterior to the palpable subclavian pulse. The needle is held between the thumb and index finger and oriented parallel to the neck and caudally. It is important to avoid any dorsomedial needle orientation.

sternocleidomastoid muscle, the clavicle, and the subclavian pulse (Fig. 11.2). The interscalene groove can be identified by placing a finger behind the sternocleidomastoid muscle and then rolling laterally. Maneuvers to help identify landmarks include asking patients to lift their head against resistance to identify the sternocleidomastoid muscle. Sniffing accentuates the scalene muscles. The groove can be followed toward the clavicle. The belly of the omohyoid muscle crosses the groove and 1 cm above the clavicle the subclavian pulse is usually palpated. The external jugular vein crosses the interscalene groove and posterior border of the sternocleidomastoid muscle at the level of the cricoid cartilage. The needle insertion site is immediately posterior to the subclavian pulse.

If the subclavian pulse is not palpable, needle insertion is 2 cm lateral to the clavicular head of the sternocleidomastoid muscle and 2 cm proximal from the clavicle. Needle insertion should be closer to the palpable middle scalene muscle than to the anterior scalene muscle because the brachial plexus lies in closer proximity to this muscle.

◈ Technique

As for all regional anesthetic procedures, after checking that emergency equipment is complete and in working order, intravenous access, ECG, pulse oximetry, and blood pressure monitoring are established. Asepsis is observed.

The patient is placed in the supine position with the head turned away from the side to be blocked. The arm is placed in view resting on the abdomen. The skin and subcutaneous tissue are infiltrated with local anesthetic. Light sedation may aid patient comfort. The subclavian artery is palpated above the medial third of the clavicle.

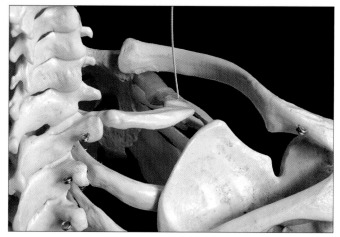

Figure 11.4 Supraclavicular block technique: deep insertion. The first rib may be contacted on deep insertion.

A 35-mm 21-G insulated needle is used. The stimulating current is set at 1 mA, 2 Hz, and 0.1 ms. Needle orientation is caudad and parallel to the neck (Fig. 11.3). It is important to avoid any dorsomedial orientation. At a depth of 1–2 cm a fascial sheath is entered. The superior trunk of the brachial plexus is usually located first. The needle position is adjusted while decreasing the current to 0.35 mA with maintenance of the muscle response.

The response that results in the greatest block success is muscle contraction below the shoulder. Responses indicating incorrect needle locations include diaphragmatic contraction (the phrenic nerve lies on the anterior scalene—too anterior a position) and contraction of the posterior compartment muscles of the shoulder (suprascapular nerve stimulation—too posterior a needle position). Contact with the first rib may occur on deep needle insertion (Fig. 11.4). The subclavian

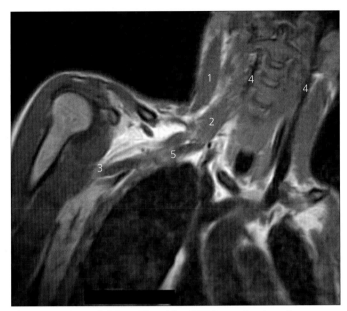

Figure 11.5 Coronal oblique T1-weighted MR image showing relevant anatomy and spread of 40 mL of contrast. Note predominantly caudad spread of contrast below the clavicle. 1, sternocleidomastoid muscle; 2, posterior and middle scalene muscles; 3, contrast spread; 4, vertebral arteries; 5, subclavian artery and brachial plexus divisions.

artery lies within the brachial plexus fascial sheath and injection in its proximity will produce successful block. If the artery is entered initially, the needle is withdrawn and oriented dorsolaterally.

Incremental injection of local anesthetic is made with repeated aspiration. For this block, 40 mL of local anesthetic is adequate (Fig. 11.5).

Continuous technique

Continuous supraclavicular block is similar to the single-shot technique. As with other continuous nerve block techniques, the initial dose of local anesthetic is usually injected and only then is the infusion of a more dilute local anesthetic initiated.

Once the local anesthetic is injected, the catheter is carefully inserted some 5 cm beyond the tip of the cannula while keeping the cannula immobile. Once the catheter is inserted, the cannula is withdrawn while simultaneously advancing the catheter to prevent its dislodgement. The catheter is secured with a transparent dressing. With this approach a 2–3-cm tunnel can also help to optimize catheter fixation. Compared with the interscalene approach, this part of the body is minimally exposed to movement, which decreases the risk of catheter displacement.

✧ Adverse effects

Pneumothorax risk is decreased by avoiding any dorsomedial needle orientation.

Local anesthetic toxicity due to intravascular injection; risk decreased by careful aspiration.

Clinical Pearls

- The plexus is closer to the middle scalene than to the anterior scalene.

- Phrenic nerve block is less likely than with the interscalene technique because here it is further away on the anterior scalene muscle.

- Infiltration of the skin and subcutaneous tissue should not be too deep because the plexus may be quite superficial.

Suggested reading

Klaastad O, Smedby O. The supraclavicular lateral para vascular approach for brachial plexus regional anesthesia: a simulation study using magnetic resonance imaging. Anesth Analg 2001; 93: 442–446.

Winnie AP. Plexus anesthesia, Vol. 1. Perivascular techniques of brachial plexus block. Copenhagen: Schultz; 1983.

CHAPTER 12
Suprascapular block

◈ Indications

Surgical—Surgical procedures on the shoulder as a supplementary analgesic technique.
Therapeutic—Shoulder pain; frozen shoulder (to facilitate physiotherapy).

◈ Contraindications

Absolute
See Chapter 4.
Relative
Hemorrhagic diathesis; anticoagulation treatment; and contralateral pneumothorax or pneumonectomy.

◈ Anatomy

The suprascapular nerve receives fibers from the fifth and sixth cervical nerve roots. It branches from the superior trunk of the brachial plexus and courses posteriorly or deep toward the scapula. It passes through the suprascapular notch under the transverse scapular ligament to enter the supraspinatus fossa. It then passes around the lateral aspect of the neck of the scapula into the infraspinous fossa. It provides sensation to the shoulder and acromioclavicular joint.

◈ Surface anatomy

The spine of the scapula is the main bony landmark for the suprascapular block (Fig. 12.1). It can be palpated from the medial aspect of the scapula and followed laterally and superiorly to the acromion. The midpoint of the spine of scapula is located and 2 cm superiorly is the needle insertion point.

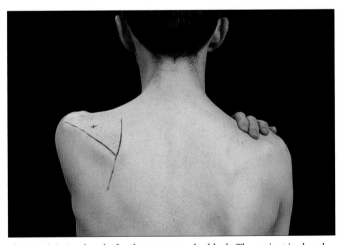

Figure 12.1 Landmarks for the suprascapular block. The patient is placed in the sitting or standing position with the hand of the side to be blocked placed on the opposite shoulder. This draws the scapula off the chest wall and decreases the risk of pneumothorax. The spine and medial border of the scapular are identified and marked. The midpoint of the spine of the scapula is located; 2 cm superiorly is the needle insertion point.

◈ Technique

As for all regional anesthetic procedures, after checking that the emergency equipment is complete and functional, intravenous access, ECG, pulse oximetry, and blood pressure monitoring are established. Asepsis is observed.

The block is performed with the patient in the sitting or standing position, with the hand of the side to be blocked resting on the contralateral shoulder (Fig. 12.2). The operator stands behind the patient. To reduce the risk of pneumothorax, as short a needle as practical is used. Needle orientation is caudad and posterior. The needle is advanced until bony contact is made, withdrawn slightly, and 10 mL of local anesthetic injected after careful aspiration (Fig. 12.3). It is not necessary to locate the scapular notch nor to elicit paresthesia because these increase the risk of pneumothorax and nerve injury.

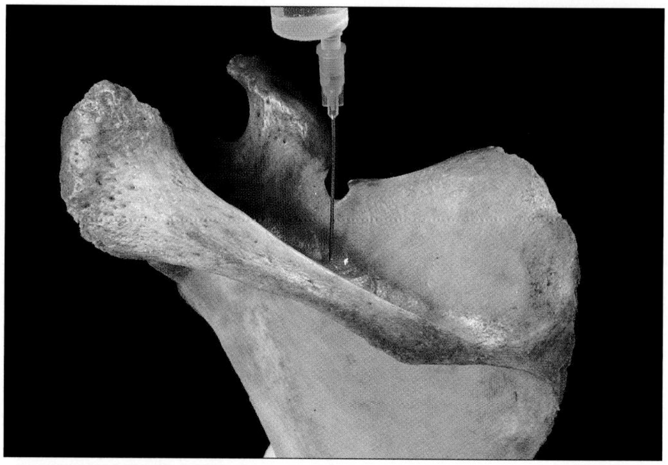

Figure 12.3 Suprascapular block technique. On bony contact the needle is withdrawn 1–2 mm and 6–8 mL of local anesthetic is injected. Note the needle does not enter the suprascapular notch.

Continuous technique

A continuous anesthesia is possible. A technique similar to the single-injection technique described can be used. An 18-G Tuohy needle is inserted caudally and posteriorly from a puncture site 2 cm cephalad from the midpoint of the spine of the scapula. On bony contact, the needle is withdrawn slightly and a catheter threaded through the needle. The needle is withdrawn while simultaneously advancing the catheter to prevent its dislodgment. The catheter is secured with a transparent dressing. The catheter can be tunneled superiorly to a non-mobile site on the back to prevent dislodgment. Patient and staff should be warned that the shoulder will be asensate during infusion. Attention should be paid to same during mobilization and physiotherapy.

◈ Adverse effects

Hematoma due to suprascapular artery or vein puncture is rare.

Pneumothorax is rare, especially if the suprascapular notch is not entered.

Clinical Pearls

• Excellent block for analgesia of the shoulder.

• Easy to learn.

Suggested reading

Wasseff MR. Suprascapular nerve block. A new approach for the management of frozen shoulder. Anesthesia 1992; 47: 120–123.

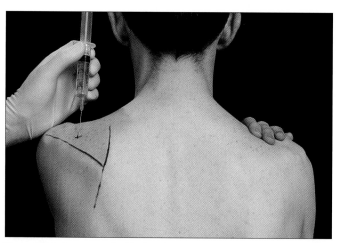

Figure 12.2 Suprascapular block technique. The needle is inserted caudally and slightly posteriorly.

CHAPTER 13
Vertical infraclavicular block

✧ Indications

Surgical—Surgical procedures at the elbow, forearm, and hand.

Therapeutic—Complex regional pain syndrome; post-amputation pain; vascular disease and injuries; tumor-related pain; prolonged postoperative analgesia (continuous technique).

✧ Contraindications

Absolute
See Chapter 4.

Relative
Hemorrhagic diathesis; anticoagulant therapy; local neural injury; risk of compartment syndrome; and distorted anatomy (due to previous surgery or trauma, e.g. fractured clavicle).

✧ Anatomy

The brachial plexus passes behind the clavicle to enter the axilla. Here it lies lateral to the subclavian vessels and dome of the lung (Fig. 13.1). Above the clavicle the trunks have formed divisions that continue to form the cords of the plexus in the axilla.

The plexus lies deep to skin, pectoralis major, and the clavipectoral fascia. The origin of the lateral cord lies most superficial. Deeper and slightly laterally, the plexus forms a

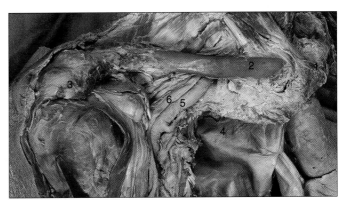

Figure 13.1 Cadaver structures illustrating anatomy pertinent to the vertical infraclavicular block technique. 1, Sternal notch; 2, clavicle; 3, anterior aspect of the acromion; 4, pleural cavity; 5, subclavian artery; 6, brachial plexus.

tight arrangement, making this site a good one for achieving a comprehensive block of the plexus. The plexus lies approximately 2–4 cm from the skin in adults.

✧ Surface anatomy

Important bony landmarks are the clavicle, anterior aspect of the acromion, the suprasternal notch, and the spine of the scapula. The distance between the suprasternal notch and anterior aspect of the acromion is measured and divided equally to find the needle insertion point, inferior to the clavicle (Fig. 13.2). Recent studies have shown that the

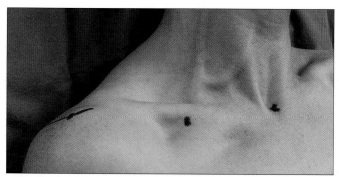

Figure 13.2 Landmarks for the vertical infraclavicular block. The suprasternal notch and anterior aspect of the acromion are marked. The measured distance between these points is divided equally to find the needle insertion point. The subclavian artery can be palpated above the clavicle and medial to the needle insertion point.

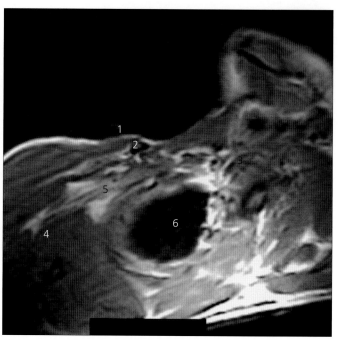

Figure 13.3 Axial oblique T1-weighted MR image showing anatomy relevant to the vertical infraclavicular block. 1, Injection point; 2, clavicle; 3, superomedial; 4, inferolateral; 5, brachial plexus; 6, apex of lung.

optimal site in females may be 0.8 cm lateral to the mid-point. In adults this distance is usually greater than 17 cm. A healed fractured clavicle will change the relations of this insertion point and is thus a relative contraindication for this block.

It may be difficult to locate the anterior aspect of the acromion. This can be facilitated by locating the spine of the scapula and tracing its border forward to the most anterior bony prominence. This point can be confirmed as the anterior prominence of the acromion by asking the patient to raise the arm. The bony prominence of the acromion will not move, unlike the head of the humerus.

The needle insertion point is lateral to the apex of the lung (Fig. 13.3). This can be confirmed by palpating the subclavian artery above the clavicle and medial to the needle insertion point.

⬦ Technique

As for all regional anesthetic procedures, after checking that emergency equipment is complete and in working order, intravenous access, ECG, pulse oximetry, and blood pressure monitoring are established. Asepsis is observed.

The patient is placed supine, with the upper arm at the side of the body and the hand resting on the abdomen; the head is rotated slightly to the opposite side. The needle insertion site is anesthetized. A 50-mm 21-G insulated needle is used. The stimulating current is set at 1 mA, 2 Hz, and 0.1 ms. The needle is advanced vertically, perpendicular to the patient trolley rather than to the chest wall (Fig. 13.4), until the appropriate muscle response is obtained. The needle position is adjusted while reducing the current to 0.35 mA with maintenance of the muscle response.

Elbow flexion (musculocutaneous nerve) is often seen first. Advancing the needle deeper and slightly laterally results in

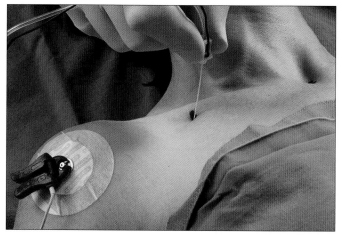

Figure 13.4 Vertical infraclavicular block technique. The needle (50 mm) is first inserted perpendicular to the patient trolley with no medial orientation.

distal muscle responses; movement of the wrist or fingers indicates an optimum needle position. Pectoralis contraction indicates too medial a needle position. Deltoid contraction is not acceptable because it is due to stimulation of the axillary nerve, which runs outside the plexus sheath.

The plexus is usually found at a depth of 2–4 cm. Incremental injection of local anesthetic is made with repeated aspiration. For this block, 40 mL of local anesthetic is sufficient (Fig. 13.5).

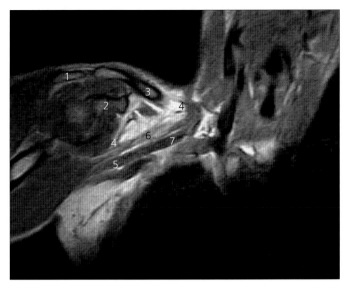

Figure 13.5 Coronal oblique T1-weighted MR image after injection of 30 mL of contrast, showing spread of contrast predominantly inferolaterally toward the axilla. Little contrast spreads superomedially. No contrast is seen above the clavicle. 1, Acromion; 2, coracoid; 3, clavicle; 4, contrast spread; 5, axillary artery; 6, brachial plexus cords; 7, subclavian artery.

Continuous technique

Continuous infraclavicular block is similar to the single-shot technique. As with other continuous nerve block techniques, the initial dose of local anesthetic is injected and only then is the infusion of a more dilute local anesthetic initiated. This facilitates block onset and catheter placement.

After the local anesthetic is injected, the catheter is carefully inserted some 5 cm beyond the tip of the cannula while keeping the cannula immobile. Once the catheter is inserted, the cannula is withdrawn while simultaneously advancing the catheter to prevent its dislodgment. The catheter is secured with a transparent dressing. With this approach a 2–3-cm tunnel medially can also help to optimize catheter fixation. This part of the body is minimally exposed to movement, which makes this block ideal for a continuous technique. Although the approach to this block is perpendicular to the plexus, catheter placement in practice is not a problem especially if a stimulating Tuohy needle is used.

Adverse effects

Unilateral paralysis of the diaphragm due to phrenic nerve block (less likely than with the supraclavicular approach).

Horner syndrome due to stellate ganglion block. These are unusual because local anesthetic rarely passes above the clavicle.

Neural injury is extremely rare.

Local anesthetic toxicity due to intravascular injection; risk decreased by avoiding medial orientation of the needle.

Pneumothorax is more likely in smaller, overweight patients. Particular attention must be paid to avoiding medial needle deviation and not using a needle greater than 50 mm in length.

Clinical Pearls

• Correct identification of the anterior aspect of the acromion is important. It is useful to follow the spine of the scapula anteriorly to the acromion. A finger resting on the acromion will not move as the patient flexes his or her shoulder.

• Practice locating this important landmark.

• If the musculocutaneous nerve is stimulated, moving the needle a little more laterally will enter the main part of the plexus.

• If the plexus is not located by 4 cm, the block should be reattempted a little more laterally (0.5–1 cm); do not move medially because this will increase the risk of vessel puncture and pneumothorax.

• This approach is excellent for a continuous technique.

Suggested reading

Greher M, Retzel G, Niel P, et al. Ultrasonographic assessment of topographic anatomy in volunteers suggests a modification of infraclavicular vertical brachial plexus block. BJA 2002; 88(5): 632–636.

Kilka HG, Geiger P, Mehrkens HH. Die vertikale infraklavikulare Blockade des Plexus brachialis. Anaesthesist 1995; 44: 339–344.

Klaastad O, Lilleas FG, Rotnes JS, et al. A magnetic resonance imaging study of modifications to the infraclavicular brachial plexus block. Anesth Analg 2000; 91: 929–933.

CHAPTER 14

Axillary block

⬧ Indications

Surgical—Surgical procedures on the forearm and hand; lower arm surgery may also require block of musculocutaneous nerve.

Therapeutic—Complex regional pain syndrome; postherpetic neuralgia; postamputation pain; vascular diseases and injuries; prolonged postoperative analgesia (continuous technique).

⬧ Contraindications

Absolute
See Chapter 4.
Relative
Hemorrhagic diathesis; anticoagulation treatment; and upper arm fractures or other conditions preventing abduction of the arm, such as frozen shoulder.

⬧ Anatomy

At the site of axillary block the terminal nerves of the brachial plexus form a particular pattern with the axillary artery (Fig. 14.1). Around the second part of the artery—the divisions being produced by the pectoralis minor muscle—the median nerve lies anteriorly, the radial nerve posteriorly, and the ulnar nerve posteromedially (Fig. 14.2). The axillary vein lies more

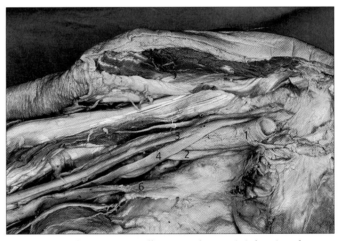

Figure 14.1 Cadaver structures illustrating characteristic location of nerves to axillary artery. 1, Axillary artery; 2, radial nerve; 3, median nerve; 4, ulnar nerve; 5, musculocutaneous nerve; 6, axillary vein.

medial. The musculocutaneous nerve has left the fascial sheath at the level of the coracoid and is thus unlikely to be anesthetized with single-injection axillary technique. The medial cutaneous nerve of arm and the intercostobrachial nerve lie subcutaneously.

⬧ Surface anatomy

For all techniques of axillary brachial plexus block, palpation of the axillary pulse is paramount. The needle insertion point

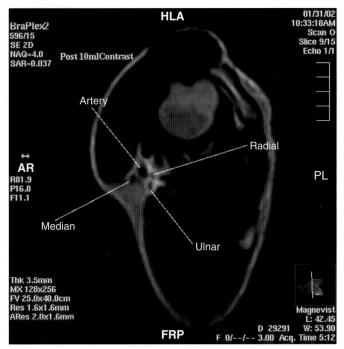

Figure 14.2 Sagittal T1-weighted MR image of axilla after injection of 10 mL of contrast, highlighting the arrangement of the nerves around the axillary artery.

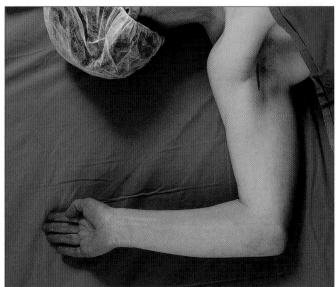

Figure 14.3 The axillary block. The patient is placed in the supine position, with the arm abducted and forearm flexed to 80° and parallel to the long axis of the body.

is located proximally along the line of the pulse. Abduction of the shoulder and flexion of the elbow bring the axilla into view. The anterior axillary fold is formed by pectoralis major muscle with the posterior axillary fold by latissimus dorsi and teres major muscles. The pulsation of the lower part of the axillary artery can be felt by palpating the medial side of the arm just in front of the posterior axillary fold. In very muscular individuals, it may be necessary to decrease the degree of abduction to palpate the artery. The pulsation is followed proximally and marked.

With single-injection techniques, it is important to identify the pulse as far proximal in the axilla as possible. This will increase the success rate for musculocutaneous nerve block with single-injection technique. The belly of the coraco-brachialis muscle should be identified because its infiltration here will block the musculocutaneous nerve.

◈ Technique

As for all regional anesthetic procedures, after checking that the emergency equipment is complete and functional, intravenous access, ECG, pulse oximetry, and blood pressure monitoring are established. Asepsis is observed.

The patient lies supine with the upper arm abducted (80°) and elbow flexed (90°) (Fig. 14.3). Hyperabduction should be avoided because it can make palpation of the artery difficult

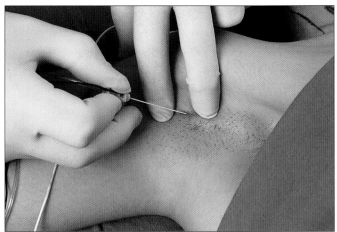

Figure 14.4 Axillary block technique. The needle is first inserted anterior to the palpable axillary pulse. The needle is oriented to follow the course of the neurovascular bundle.

and distort the distribution of local anesthetic. The axillary artery is palpated as proximally as possible under the lateral edge of the pectoralis major muscle, and fixed with the index and middle fingers. A 35-mm 21-G insulated stimulating needle is used. The stimulating current is set at 1.0 mA, 2 Hz, and 0.1 ms. The needle is advanced proximally at an angle of 30° in the direction (Fig. 14.4) of the neurovascular sheath. Entry of the needle into the neurovascular sheath is confirmed by a 'fascial click'. The needle is advanced slowly until the appropriate muscle response is obtained.

Stimulation of the median nerve produces flexion of the middle and index fingers, thumb, and pronation and flexion of the wrist. Stimulation of the ulnar nerve produces flexion of

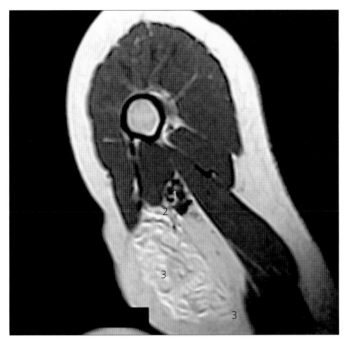

Figure 14.5 Axial oblique T1-weighted MR image showing spread of contrast outside and away from the axillary sheath. This followed excellent median nerve stimulation down to 0.5 mA and insertion of catheter. This suggests that perhaps 0.5 mA is too high a current to be sure that the needle is inside the axillary sheath. 1, Brachial plexus and axillary vessels; 2, nerve sheath; 3, contrast spread.

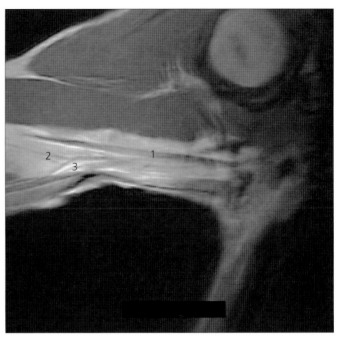

Figure 14.6 Coronal T1-weighted MR image after injection of 40 mL of contrast. Injection was made without distal pressure being applied. 1, Profunda brachii artery; 2, radial nerve; 3, median nerve.

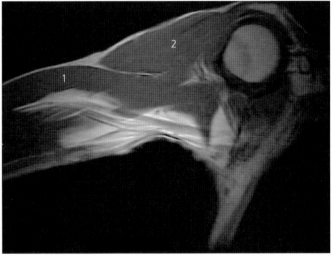

Figure 14.7 Coronal T1-weighted MR image 30 min post injection of 40 mL of contrast. Note spread is almost entirely away from the axilla, two-thirds of the length of the upper arm. 1, Biceps muscle; 2, deltoid muscle.

the ring and little fingers with ulnar deviation of the wrist, while stimulation of the radial nerve will produce dorsiflexion of the fingers and wrist. Finger flexion alone in the case of the ring and little fingers could represent either ulnar or median stimulation. The needle position is adjusted while decreasing the current to 0.30 mA with maintenance of the muscle response (Fig. 14.5). A muscle response in the upper arm should not be accepted. Individual nerves can be targeted and located with ease. Ideally the nerve(s) supplying the area of surgery should be sought.

Incremental injection of the local anesthetic is made with repeated aspiration. To block terminal nerves of the plexus, 40 mL of local anesthetic is sufficient. If a multiple-injection technique is used, 10 mL at each site is adequate. The stimulating current needs to be increased for the second and subsequent nerves because the previously injected local anesthetic will increase the electrical resistance in the area. To increase the likelihood of blocking the musculocutaneous nerve, digital pressure is maintained distal to the site of injection to encourage proximal spread of the local anesthetic within the axillary sheath; a tourniquet may be used for a similar effect (Figs 14.6, 14.7). The arm is then placed across the chest.

If an upper arm tourniquet is to be used, additional block of the intercostobrachial nerve and medial cutaneous nerve of arm is of value to reduce the cutaneous element of the pain due to the tourniquet. The intercostobrachial nerve is the lateral cutaneous branch of the second intercostal nerve. The medial cutaneous nerve of arm originates from the medial cord of the brachial plexus. Block of both nerves can be achieved with a subcutaneous injection of local anesthetic in the medial aspect of the upper arm (Fig. 14.8). Injection should be made from the biceps muscle to the triceps muscle.

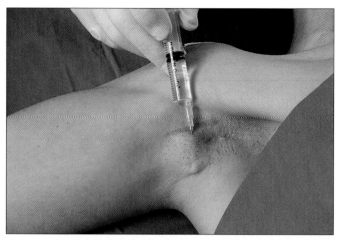

Figure 14.8 Intercostobrachial block technique. A subcutaneous injection (5–6 mL) in the axilla will anesthetize the intercostobrachial and medial cutaneous nerve of arm.

Musculocutaneous nerve block

The musculocutaneous nerve (C5, 6) is a branch of the lateral cord of the brachial plexus. It leaves the plexus fascial sheath at the level of the coracoid process, pierces the coraco-brachialis muscle, and then runs between the biceps and brachialis muscles in the arm. It passes through the antecubital fossa deep to the biceps tendon and continues as the lateral cutaneous nerve of the forearm. It supplies motor fibers to the coracobrachialis muscle, the biceps muscle, and brachialis muscles. It is the sensory supply of the skin covering the radial aspect of the lower two-thirds of the forearm.

The musculocutaneous nerve can be blocked as part of an infraclavicular technique using the vertical infraclavicular or coracoid approaches (cf. Ch. 13). An injection into the body of coracobrachialis will also anesthetize it without the need to elicit paresthesia or a motor response. It can be blocked as part of the midhumeral approach (cf. Ch. 15). The lateral cutaneous nerve of arm can be blocked at the elbow by an injection just lateral to the tendon of biceps at the elbow crease. A 23-G needle is inserted to a depth of 2–3 cm and injection of 4 mL of local anesthetic is made.

Continuous technique

Generally, catheters placed by the axillary route are easily displaced. Nevertheless, the axillary brachial plexus block is the most widely used continuous technique. With this block the approach is parallel to the neurovascular bundle, which facilitates catheter placement. Tunneling is recommended. As with the single-injection technique, the musculocutaneous nerve is frequently not anesthetized.

◈ Adverse effects

Hematoma formation due to puncture of the axillary artery.

Neural injuries are extremely rare.

Local anesthetic toxicity is a particular risk because intravascular injection into the axillary vessels is possible.

Traumatic pseudoaneurysm may be accompanied by post-operative paresthesia and plexus paralysis.

Clinical Pearls

- Palpate axillary artery as high in the axilla as possible.
- Check site of surgery and target the relevant nerve.
- Distal pressure increases chance of blocking musculocutaneous nerve.
- To confirm median nerve stimulation palpate flexor carpi radialis tendon.
- Be prepared to do 'escape blocks' at elbow or wrist or midhumeral.

Suggested reading

Bouaziz H, Narchi P, Mercier FJ, et al. The use of a selective axillary nerve block for outpatient hand surgery. Anesth Analg 1998; 86: 746–748.

Finucane BT, Yilling F. Safety of supplementing axillary brachial plexus blocks. Anesthesiology 1989; 70: 401–403.

Klaastad O, Smedby O, Thompson GE, et al. Distribution of local anesthetic in axillary brachial plexus block: a clinical and magnetic resonance imaging study. Anesthesiology 2002; 96: 1315–1324.

Lavoie J, Martin R, Tetrault JP, et al. Axillary plexus block using a peripheral nerve stimulator: single or multiple injections. Can J Anaesth 1992; 39: 583–586.

Patridge BL, Katz J, Benirshoke K. Functional anatomy of the brachial plexus sheath: implications for anesthesia. Anesthesiology 1987; 66: 743–747.

Vester-Andersen T, Christiansen C, Sorensen M, et al. Perivascular axillary block II: influence of volume of local anesthetic on neural blockade. Acta Anaesthesiol Scand 1983; 27: 95–98.

CHAPTER 15
Midhumeral block

Indications

Surgical—Surgical procedures in the innervated area; supplementation of incomplete anesthesia of the brachial plexus.
Therapeutic—Complex regional pain syndrome; postherpetic neuralgia; postamputation pain; prolonged postoperative analgesia (continuous technique).

Contraindications

Absolute
See Chapter 4.
Relative
Hemorrhagic diathesis; anticoagulation treatment; and local neural injury.

Anatomy

The humeral canal, containing the terminal nerves of the brachial plexus and the brachial artery, lies on the medial aspect of the arm. At this location it is possible to anesthetize the four major nerves of the upper limb separately. The humeral canal is bounded superiorly by the biceps muscle, inferiorly by triceps, laterally by coracobrachialis, and medially by skin and subcutaneous tissue. The needle insertion site is at the junction between the upper one-third and the lower two-thirds of the humerus, in proximity to the brachial artery. A common mistake is to choose a needle insertion site at the midpoint of the humerus. Here the radial nerve is inaccessible because it lies in the radial groove on the posterior aspect of the humerus. At the needle insertion site, the four major nerves of the upper limb have a characteristic location in relation to the brachial artery. The median nerves lies anterior to the artery, the ulnar nerve posteromedially, and the radial nerve posteriorly adjacent to the humerus. The musculocutaneous nerve lies superior to the artery and under biceps at this point. The medial cutaneous nerve of the arm lies medial to the artery within the canal.

Surface anatomy

The main landmarks for the midhumeral block include the junction between the upper one-third and lower two-thirds of the humerus and the brachial artery. This can be approximated as three fingers' breadth below the anterior axillary fold (Fig. 15.1).

Technique

As for all regional anesthetic procedures, after checking that emergency equipment is complete and in working order, intravenous access, ECG, pulse oximetry, and blood pressure monitoring are established. Asepsis is observed.

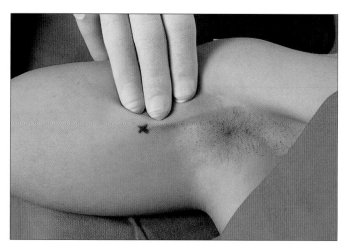

Figure 15.1 Landmarks for the midhumeral block. The needle insertion point for the midhumeral block is located at the junction between the upper third and lower two-thirds of the humerus. This can be approximated as three fingers' breadth below the anterior axillary fold.

The arm of the patient is placed at right angles to the body, with the forearm extended and supine. At the junction between the upper and middle thirds of the arm, a line is drawn over the brachial artery. The needle insertion point is infiltrated with local anesthetic using a 25-G needle. A 50-mm 22-G insulated needle connected to a peripheral nerve stimulator is inserted almost tangentially to the skin, between the brachial artery and the palpating finger, in the direction of the axilla, in order to locate the median nerve (Fig. 15.2). The stimulating current is set at 1.0 mA, 2 Hz, and 0.1 ms. The needle is advanced slowly until the appropriate muscle response is obtained. The needle position is adjusted while

decreasing the current to 0.35 mA with maintenance of the muscle response. Stimulation of the median nerve will produce contraction of the flexor carpi radialis and flexor digitorum superficialis of the fingers. Incremental injections of local anesthetic (6–8 mL) are made with repeated aspiration.

After blocking the median nerve, the current is increased to 2 mA, and the needle withdrawn and redirected beneath and medial to the artery (Fig. 15.3). Stimulation of the ulnar nerve induces contraction of the flexor carpi ulnaris muscle. Incremental injection of local anesthetic (6–8 mL) is made with repeated aspiration.

The needle is now withdrawn and, with a high level of stimulation in the subcutaneous position, redirected toward the radial nerve. This nerve is posterior to the artery, close to the humerus (Fig. 15.4). Stimulation of the radial nerve causes contraction of the extensor muscles of the forearm. Incremental injections of local anesthetic (6–8 mL) are made with repeated aspiration.

To block the musculocutaneous nerve, the needle is directed from its initial subcutaneous position beneath the biceps muscle (Fig. 15.5). Stimulation of this nerve induces contraction of the biceps muscle and flexion of the elbow. Incremental injections of local anesthetic (6 mL) are made with repeated aspiration. A final 3 mL is injected medial to the artery to block the medial cutaneous nerves of the arm and the forearm.

Continuous technique

Continuous midhumeral techniques have not been described, but it may be possible to provide continuous anesthesia of an individual upper arm nerve at this location.

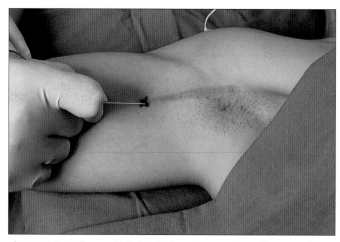

Figure 15.2 Midhumeral block technique: locating the median nerve. The needle is inserted anterior and parallel to the brachial pulse to locate the median nerve.

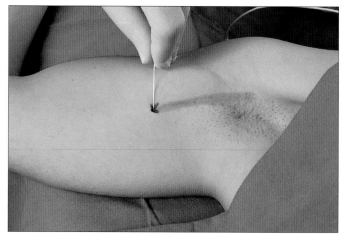

Figure 15.3 Midhumeral block technique: locating the ulnar nerve. The needle is inserted medial and perpendicular to the brachial pulse to locate the ulnar nerve.

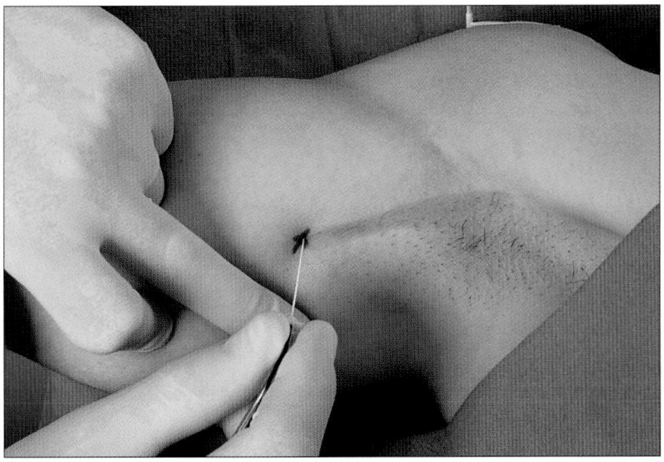

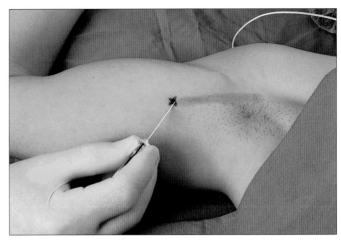

Figure 15.4 Midhumeral block technique: locating the radial nerve. The skin is retracted inferior to the brachial pulse and oriented perpendicular to the artery and toward the humerus to locate the radial nerve.

Figure 15.5 Midhumeral block technique: locating the musculocutaneous nerve. The needle is inserted superior to the brachial pulse and under biceps to locate the musculocutaneous nerve.

Adverse effects

Hematoma formation due to puncture of the brachial artery.

Neural injuries are extremely rare.

Local anesthetic toxicity due to intravascular injection into the brachial vessels leading rapidly to toxic reactions. Over-dosage or intravascular diffusion can also cause symptoms of local anesthetic toxicity. Slow injection of local anesthetics will decrease the incidence of this complication.

Pseudoaneurysm may be accompanied by postoperative paresthesia.

Suggested reading

Bouaziz H, Narchi P, Mercier FJ, et al. Comparison between conventional axillary block and a new approach at the midhumeral level. Anesth Analg 1997; 84: 1058–1067.

Frizelle HP. Technical note: the humeral canal approach to the brachial plexus. Yale J Biol Med 1998; 71: 585–589.

Hickey RM, Hoffman J, Tingle LJ, et al. Comparison of the clinical efficacy of three perivascular techniques for axillary brachial plexus block. Reg Anesth 1993; 18: 335–338.

Clinical Pearls

• Sedation is paramount with this multi-injection technique.

• Palpation of the brachial artery must be performed with care. The palpating finger may approximate the needle tip to the nerve while in fact it is further away. Thus final needle location and injection must be performed without digital palpation of the artery.

• Often differentiation between median and ulnar nerve on muscular contraction is difficult. By resting the hand on the forearm it is easy to distinguish between contraction of flexor carpi radialis (median) and flexor carpi ulnaris (ulnar). This may be due to Martin–Gruber anastomosis—communication of the median and ulnar nerves in the arm and forearm.

CHAPTER 16
Elbow blocks

Indications

Surgical—Surgical procedures in the innervated area; supplementation of incomplete anesthesia of the brachial plexus.
Therapeutic—None.

Contraindications

Absolute
See Chapter 4.
Relative
Hemorrhagic diathesis; anticoagulation treatment; local neural injury; and distorted anatomy (due to previous surgery or trauma).

Anatomy

The three major nerves of the forearm can be blocked at the elbow (Fig. 16.1), and also the three cutaneous nerves of the forearm.

The *median nerve*, which lies anteromedially to the brachial artery near the axilla, crosses medial to the artery in the arm. At the elbow it lies between the tendons of brachialis and pronator teres, and deep to the bicipital aponeurosis. It passes between both heads of pronator teres to enter the forearm (Fig. 16.2). The median nerve provides sensory innervation to the lateral half of the palm, flexor aspect of the thumb, index finger, middle finger, and radial side of the ring finger.

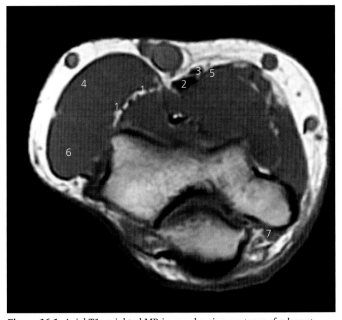

Figure 16.1 Axial T1-weighted MR image showing anatomy of relevant structures at the elbow. 1, Radial nerve with profunda brachii artery and vein; 2, biceps tendon; 3, brachial artery; 4, brachioradialis; 5, site of median nerve; 6, extensor carpi radialis longus; 7, ulnar nerve.

The *radial nerve* passes between the long and medial head of triceps to travel around the humerus and emerges on the anterior aspect of the arm above brachioradialis. It passes deep to brachioradialis over the lateral epicondyle, where it divides into a deep and a superficial branch (Fig. 16.2). The radial nerve

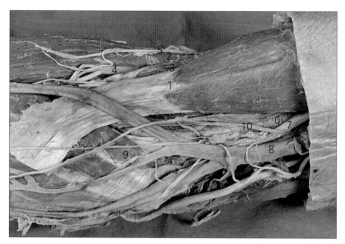

Figure 16.2 Cadaver structures illustrating anatomy pertinent to median and radial nerve block at the elbow. 1, Biceps muscle and aponeurosis; 2, brachioradialis; 3, brachialis; 4, radial nerve; 5, lateral cutaneous nerve of forearm; 6, brachial artery; 7, median nerve; 8, brachial vein; 9, pronator teres; 10, medial cutaneous nerve of forearm.

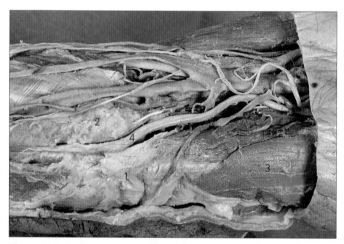

Figure 16.3 Cadaver structures illustrating anatomy pertinent to ulnar nerve block at the elbow. 1, Olecranon process; 2, medial epicondyle; 3, triceps muscle; 4, ulnar nerve.

provides sensation for the radial half of the dorsum of the hand, the back of the thumb, and part of the back of the index finger.

The *ulnar nerve* leaves the brachial artery halfway down the arm and passes behind the medial epicondyle in a fibrous tunnel. It passes between the two heads of flexor carpi ulnaris to enter the forearm (Fig. 16.3). The ulnar nerve provides sensation for the ulnar half of the dorsum of the hand, little finger, and ulnar side of the ring finger.

Surface anatomy

Important structures include the medial and lateral epicondyles of the humerus, olecranon process, intercondylar

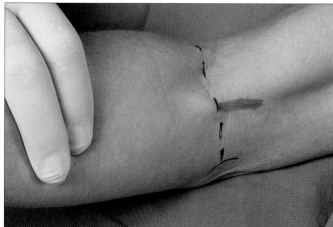

Figure 16.4 Landmarks for nerve blocks at the elbow. Landmarks include the medial and lateral epicondyles of the humerus, intercondylar skin crease, biceps tendon, brachioradialis muscle, and brachial pulse. The biceps tendon can be palpated with elbow flexion beneath the intercondylar crease and it runs laterally to the head of the radius. The brachioradialis muscle can be palpated lateral to the biceps tendon. The brachial artery is palpated medial to the biceps muscle.

skin crease, biceps tendon, brachioradialis muscle, and brachial artery (Fig. 16.4). The biceps tendon can be palpated with elbow flexion beneath the intercondylar crease, and it runs laterally to the head of the radius. The brachioradialis muscle can be palpated lateral to the biceps tendon. The brachial artery is palpated medial to the biceps muscle.

Technique

As for all regional anesthetic procedures, after checking that the emergency equipment is complete and in working order, intravenous access, ECG, pulse oximetry, and blood pressure monitoring are established. Asepsis is observed.

The patient is placed in the supine position with the arm to be blocked abducted 30° with the elbow extended on an arm board. The operator sits at the side to be blocked below the patient's elbow. The needle insertion point is infiltrated with local anesthetic using a 25-G needle. For block at the elbow, a 25-mm insulated needle is used.

Median nerve block

Needle insertion for median nerve block is medial to the brachial pulse at the level of the intercondylar crease (Fig. 16.5). Needle orientation is cephalad and toward the humerus. The stimulating current is set at 1.0 mA, 2 Hz, and 0.1 ms. The needle is advanced slowly until the appropriate muscle response is obtained: finger rather than wrist flexion. A loss of resistance is felt as the bicipital aponeurosis is punctured. The needle position is adjusted while

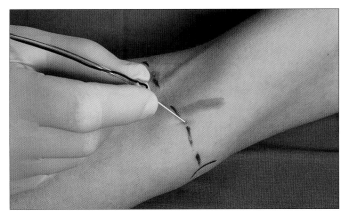

Figure 16.5 Median nerve block technique. Needle insertion for median nerve block is medial to the brachial pulse at the level of the intercondylar crease. Needle orientation is cephalad and toward the humerus.

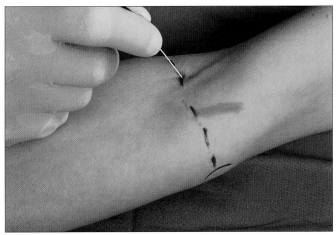

Figure 16.6 Radial nerve block technique. Needle insertion for radial nerve block is halfway between the biceps tendon and lateral border of the arm (or 1 cm lateral to the biceps tendon), in the gutter between the biceps tendon and brachioradialis at the level of the intercondylar skin crease. Needle orientation is cephalad and toward the humerus.

decreasing the current to 0.35 mA with maintenance of the muscle response. Wrist flexion may be due to direct muscle stimulation. Incremental injections of local anesthetic (4–6 mL) are made with repeated aspiration. If no twitch is found, 'walk' the needle in a medial to lateral plane.

Radial nerve block

Needle insertion for radial nerve block is halfway between the biceps tendon and lateral border of the arm (or 1 cm lateral to the biceps tendon), in the gutter between the biceps tendon and brachioradialis at the level of the intercondylar skin crease (Fig. 16.6). Needle orientation is cephalad and aimed toward the humerus (toward the lateral epicondyle). At a depth of 2–3 cm the radial nerve will be encountered. Finger and thumb extension, rather than wrist extension due to possible direct stimulation of extensor carpi radialis, results in greatest block success. Incremental injections of local anesthetic (4–6 mL) are made with repeated aspiration.

If direct brachioradialis contraction is elicited, move the needle slightly more medially. Failure to elicit an appropriate muscle response should be followed by walking the needle in a medial to lateral orientation.

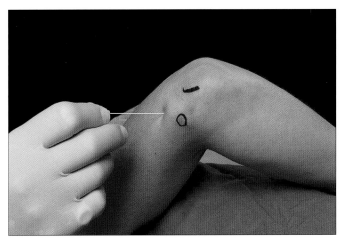

Figure 16.7 Ulnar nerve block technique. The elbow is flexed 30° and the arm internally rotated across the upper body for ulnar nerve block. Needle orientation is 45° to the skin in a cephalad direction.

Ulnar nerve block

The elbow is flexed 30° and the arm internally rotated across the upper body for ulnar nerve block. Needle orientation is 45° to the skin in a cephalad direction (Fig. 16.7). The ulnar nerve is very superficial and contacted within 0.5–1 cm. Little finger flexion and ulnar deviation of the hand, rather than wrist flexion due to possible direct flexor carpi ulnaris stimulation, results in greatest block success. Incremental injections of local anesthetic (4 mL) are made with repeated aspiration. The needle is walked in a medial to lateral direction if the ulnar

nerve is not stimulated. With elbow flexion the ulnar nerve may slip over the medial epicondyle.

Cutaneous nerves of forearm blocks

Because the branches of the sensory nerves of the forearm have already ramified extensively and cross the joint superficially in a diffuse subcutaneous network, good anesthesia of the forearm itself is difficult to obtain. The lateral cutaneous nerve of forearm can be blocked by injection deep to fascia in the muscular groove between biceps and brachioradialis. The medial cutaneous nerve of forearm can be blocked by subcutaneous injection in the intermuscular groove between biceps and pronator teres. The posterior cutaneous nerve of forearm can be blocked by subcutaneous injection from the lateral epicondyle to the olecranon.

◈ Adverse effects

Hematoma.

Neural injuries are extremely rare.

Local anesthetic toxicity due to intravascular injection, diffusion, or overdosage can cause symptoms of CNS toxicity. Slow injection of local anesthetic and repeated aspiration will decrease the incidence of this complication.

Clinical Pearls

• If a tourniquet is used then the medial cutaneous nerve of the arm needs to be blocked.

• Unlike wrist blocks, blockade at the elbow will provide good motor block in the wrist and fingers.

Suggested reading

Amoiridis G, Vlachonikolis IG. Verification of the median-to-ulnar and ulnar-to-median nerve motor fiber anastomosis in the forearm: an electrophysiological study. Clin Neurophysiol 2003; 114: 94–98.

CHAPTER 17

Wrist blocks

◈ Indications

Surgical—Hand or finger surgery not requiring a tourniquet; supplementation of incomplete brachial plexus block.
Therapeutic—Differentiation of finger or hand pain.

◈ Contraindications

Absolute
See Chapter 4.
Relative
Local neural injury and distorted anatomy (due to previous surgery or trauma).

◈ Anatomy

The hand is innervated by the three nerves that pass through the wrist (Fig. 17.1).

The *median nerve* approaches the wrist between palmaris longus (if present) and flexor carpi radialis. It can also lie beneath palmaris longus (Fig. 17.2). The median nerve provides sensation to the lateral half of the palm, flexor aspect of the thumb, index finger, middle finger, and radial side of the ring finger.

The *ulnar nerve*, in the middle of the forearm between the flexor digitorum profundus and the flexor carpi ulnaris, gives off a dorsal and a ventral cutaneous branch. At the wrist, the

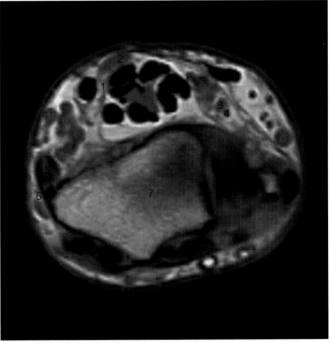

Figure 17.1 Axial MR image showing anatomy of relevant structures at the wrist. 1, Median nerve; 2, palmaris longus tendon; 3, ulnar artery; 4, ulnar nerve; 5, radial artery; 6, radial nerve; 7, radius.

ulnar nerve lies between the ulnar artery and deep to the radial border of flexor carpi ulnaris (Fig. 17.2), which inserts on the pisiform bone. Near the pisiform bone, it passes superficial to the flexor retinaculum and ends by dividing into

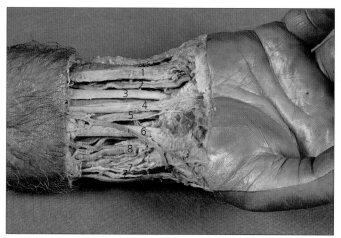

Figure 17.2 Cadaver structures illustrating anatomy pertinent to nerve blocks at the wrist. 1, Flexor carpi ulnaris; 2, ulnar nerve and artery; 3, flexor digitorum superficialis; 4, palmaris longus; 5, median nerve; 6, flexor carpi radialis; 7, superficial branches of the radial nerve; 8, radial artery.

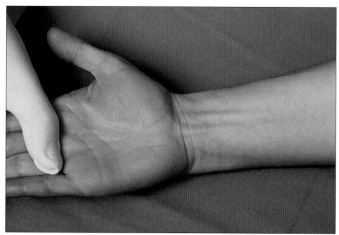

Figure 17.4 Landmarks for the nerve blocks at the wrist. Landmarks include radial and ulnar styloids, flexor carpi radialis and ulnaris, palmaris longus, radial and ulnar arteries, and the wrist skin crease.

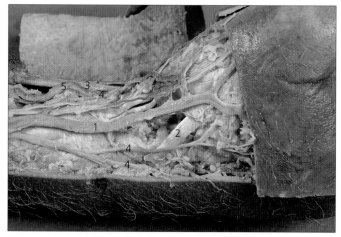

Figure 17.3 Cadaver structures illustrating anatomy pertinent to radial nerve block at the wrist. 1, Cephalic vein; 2, extensor pollicis longus; 3, flexor carpi radialis; 4, superficial branches of the radial nerve; 5, radial artery.

superficial and deep branches. The ulnar nerve provides sensation for the ulnar half of the back and front of the hand, little finger, and ulnar side of the ring finger.

The *radial nerve* at the wrist lies between the flexor carpi radialis and the radial artery (Fig. 17.3). The radial nerve provides sensation for the radial half of the back of the hand, back of the thumb, and part of the back of the index finger.

Surface anatomy

Bony landmarks include the ulnar styloid and the radial styloid carpal bones. Other landmarks include the wrist crease, flexor

carpi radialis, palmaris longus, and flexor carpi ulnaris tendons (Fig. 17.4). These tendons can be accentuated by having the patient flex the wrist while making a fist. The radial artery can be palpated lateral to the tendon of flexor carpi radialis, and the ulnar artery lateral to flexor carpi ulnaris tendon.

Technique

As for all regional anesthetic procedures, after checking that emergency equipment is complete and in working order, intravenous access, ECG, pulse oximetry, and blood pressure monitoring are established. Asepsis is observed.

The patient is placed in the supine position, with the arm abducted and extended at the elbow and wrist joints and placed on an arm board or on the operator's knee with the wrist slightly dorsiflexed. The operator sits facing the patient's hand. A paresthesia technique is the technique described here. A 15-mm 25-G needle is used.

Median nerve block

Needle insertion for median nerve block is 2 cm cephalad from the wrist crease between the tendons of flexor carpi radialis and palmaris longus, if present (Fig. 17.5). The needle and syringe are held like a pencil between the thumb and index fingers, with a cephalad needle orientation.

The patient is instructed to indicate when they feel a paresthesia in the palm and fingers. On obtaining a paresthesia the needle is withdrawn slightly. Absence of paresthesia is checked prior to injecting 3 mL of local anesthetic. A subcutaneous injection is also made on withdrawal to block the palmar cutaneous branch of the median nerve. The median

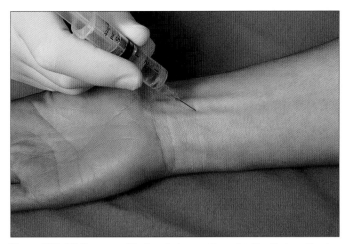

Figure 17.5 Median nerve block technique at the wrist. Needle insertion is 2 cm cephalad from the wrist crease between the tendons of flexor carpi radialis and palmaris longus (if present). The needle and syringe are held like a pencil between the thumb and index fingers, with a cephalad needle orientation.

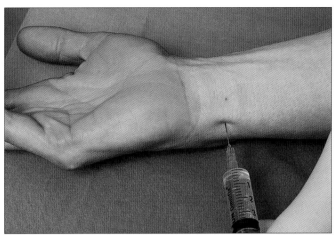

Figure 17.7 Ulnar nerve block technique at the wrist: medial approach. Needle insertion is 2 cm cephalad from the wrist crease, medial, and deep to flexor carpi ulnaris.

nerve may also be blocked by injection deep in the flexor retinaculum in the wrist.

Ulnar nerve block

Needle insertion for ulnar nerve block is 2 cm cephalad from the wrist crease lateral to flexor carpi ulnaris or medial to the tendon. For ulnar nerve block, ventral and medial approaches can be used. The needle and syringe are held like a pencil between the thumb and index fingers; needle orientation is cephalad for the ventral approach (Fig. 17.6).

The patient is instructed to indicate when they feel a paresthesia in the palm and fingers. On obtaining a paresthesia

the needle is withdrawn slightly. Absence of paresthesia is checked prior to injecting 3 mL of local anesthetic. The ulnar nerve at the wrist may also be blocked by injection medial and deep to flexor carpi ulnaris (Fig. 17.7). The medial approach is preferable because ulnar artery damage is less likely and both dorsal and palmar cutaneous branches may be blocked from the same needle insertion point.

The ulnar nerve can also be blocked 6 cm cephalad from the proximal wrist crease by injection of 4 mL of local anesthetic beneath the tendon of flexor carpi ulnaris. This method will block the dorsal and ventral branches of the ulnar nerve, and is the method of choice if anesthesia is required on the dorsal aspect of the little finger.

Radial nerve block

Needle insertion for radial nerve block is at the level of the wrist crease (Fig. 17.8). For radial nerve block at the wrist, a 30-mm 22-G needle is used. A subcutaneous injection is made from the radial styloid across the tendon of extensor pollicis brevis to the middle of the dorsal surface of the wrist (Fig. 17.9). The needle is redirected, infiltrating now across the tendon of extensor pollicis brevis to the ventral surface of the wrist and over the radial artery. A paresthesia is not sought because the radial nerve is now superficial fibers only. Local anesthetic solution is massaged in to improve the subcutaneous spread. Local anesthetic (8–10 mL) is injected.

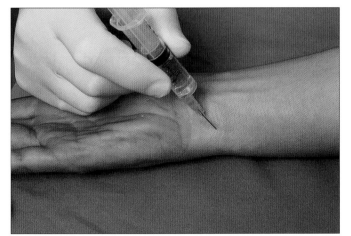

Figure 17.6 Ulnar nerve block technique at the wrist: ventral approach. Needle insertion is 2 cm cephalad from the wrist crease lateral to flexor carpi ulnaris. The needle and syringe are held like a pencil between the thumb and index fingers; needle orientation is cephalad.

⬦ Adverse effects

Hematoma.
    Neural injuries are extremely rare.

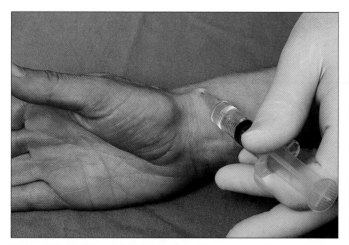

Figure 17.8 Radial nerve block technique at the wrist: needle insertion. Needle insertion is at the level of the wrist crease. A subcutaneous injection is made from the radial styloid across the tendon of extensor pollicis longus.

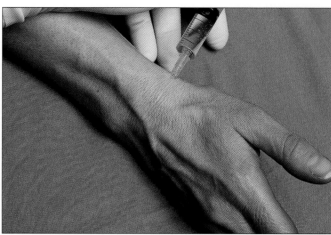

Figure 17.9 Radial nerve block technique at the wrist: subcutaneous injection. The subcutaneous injection is continued to the dorsal surface of the wrist.

Clinical Pearls

- The injection should be immediately stopped if the patient reports pain on injection or if resistance to injection is met.

- Block of radial nerve is the least consistent because this is a sensory nerve with variable subcutaneous course; thus larger volumes (10 mL) of local anesthetic are required to ensure its blockade.

- The intensity of the sensory blocks can be tested by using ice. The ulnar territory is tested on the medial aspect of the hand; the median territory on the lateral aspect of the palm at the level of the index finger; and the musculocutaneous territory on the lateral aspect of the wrist.

Suggested reading

Gebhard RE, Al-Samsam T, Greger J, et al. Distal nerve blocks at the wrist for outpatient carpal tunnel surgery offer intraoperative cardiovascular stability and reduce discharge time. Anesth Analg 2002; 95: 351–355.

Klezl Z, Krejca M, Simcik J. Role of sensory innervation variations for wrist block anesthesia. Arch Med Res 2001; 32: 155–158.

Thompson WL, Malchow RJ. Peripheral nerve blocks and anesthesia of the hand. Mil Med 2002; 167: 478–482.

CHAPTER 18

Lumbar and sacral plexus anatomy

The anterior divisions of the lumbar, sacral, and coccygeal nerves form the lumbosacral plexus. The plexus is usually divided into three parts: the lumbar, sacral, and pudendal plexuses for ease of description. The lumbar plexus primarily innervates the ventral aspect, whereas the sacral plexus innervates the dorsal aspect of the lower limb.

LUMBAR PLEXUS

The lumbar plexus (Fig. 18.1) lies deep within the psoas major muscle in front of the transverse processes of the lumbar vertebrae. It is formed by the ventral rami of the first three lumbar nerves and the greater part of the ventral ramus of the fourth nerve. All the branches of the plexus emerge from the substance of psoas major.

The first lumbar nerve, frequently supplemented by the 12th thoracic, splits into an upper and a lower branch; the upper and larger branch divides into the iliohypogastric and ilioinguinal nerves, the lower and smaller branch unites with a branch of the second lumbar to form the genitofemoral nerve.

The remainder of the second nerve, and the third and fourth nerves, divide into ventral and dorsal divisions. The ventral division of the second unites with the ventral divisions of the third and fourth nerves to form the obturator nerve. The dorsal divisions of the second and third nerves divide into two branches, a smaller branch from each uniting to form the lateral cutaneous nerve of thigh, and a larger branch from each joining with the dorsal division of the fourth nerve to form the femoral nerve.

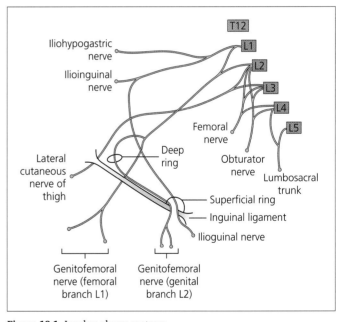

Figure 18.1 Lumbar plexus anatomy.

The iliohypogastric and ilioinguinal nerves

The iliohypogastric (L1) and ilioinguinal (L1) nerves emerge from the upper part of the lateral border of the psoas major muscle, initially together or separate throughout, with the former above the latter. They both pass laterally in front of quadratus lumborum to enter the neurovascular plane between transverse abdominis and internal oblique muscles.

The *iliohypogastric nerve* pierces internal oblique about 2 cm medial to the anterior superior iliac spine and goes on to pierce external oblique about 3 cm above the superficial inguinal ring. It supplies sensation to suprapubic skin; a lateral cutaneous branch supplies posterolateral gluteal skin.

The *ilioinguinal nerve* pierces the lower border of the internal oblique to enter the inguinal canal, which it leaves through the superficial ring to supply the skin of the anterior scrotum (mons pubis and labium majus), root of penis (clitoris), and upper medial thigh.

The lateral cutaneous nerve of thigh

The lateral cutaneous nerve of thigh (lateral femoral cutaneous nerve) arises from the dorsal divisions of the second and third lumbar nerves. It emerges from the lateral border of the psoas major about its middle, and crosses the iliacus muscle obliquely toward the anterior superior iliac spine. It passes under the inguinal ligament and over the sartorius muscle into the thigh, where it divides into two branches.

The anterior branch becomes superficial about 10 cm below the inguinal ligament and divides into branches, which are distributed to the skin of the anterior and lateral parts of the thigh as far as the knee. The posterior branch pierces the fascia lata and subdivides into branches, which pass backward across the lateral and posterior surfaces of the thigh, supplying the skin from the level of the greater trochanter to the middle of the thigh.

The femoral nerve

The femoral nerve, the largest branch of the lumbar plexus, arises from the dorsal divisions of the second, third, and fourth lumbar nerves. It descends through the fibers of the psoas major, emerging from the muscle at the lower part of its lateral border, and passes down between it and the iliacus muscle, behind the iliac fascia; it then runs beneath the inguinal ligament into the thigh, and splits into an anterior and a posterior division. Under the inguinal ligament, it is separated from the femoral artery by a portion of the psoas major. In the thigh, the anterior division of the femoral nerve gives off anterior cutaneous and muscular branches. The anterior cutaneous branches comprise the intermediate and medial cutaneous nerves.

The intermediate cutaneous nerve pierces the fascia lata (and generally the sartorius) about 7.5 cm below the inguinal ligament, and divides into two branches that descend in immediate proximity along the forepart of the thigh to supply the skin as low as the front of the knee.

The medial cutaneous nerve passes obliquely across the upper part of the sheath of the femoral artery, and divides in front or at the medial side of that vessel into two branches: an anterior and a posterior. The anterior branch runs downward on the sartorius, perforates the fascia lata at the lower third of the thigh, and divides into two branches. The posterior branch descends along the medial border of the sartorius muscle to the knee, where it pierces the fascia lata, communicates with the saphenous nerve, and gives off several cutaneous branches.

The saphenous nerve

The saphenous nerve is the largest cutaneous branch of the femoral nerve. It approaches the femoral artery where this vessel passes beneath the sartorius, and lies in front of it, behind the aponeurotic covering of the adductor canal, as far as the opening in the lower part of the adductor magnus. Here it leaves the artery and emerges from behind the lower edge of the aponeurotic covering of the canal; it descends vertically along the medial side of the knee behind the sartorius, pierces the fascia lata between the tendons of the sartorius and gracilis, and becomes subcutaneous.

The nerve then passes along the tibial side of the leg, accompanied by the great saphenous vein, descends behind the medial border of the tibia, and at the lower third of the leg divides into two branches; one continues its course along the margin of the tibia and ends at the ankle, the other passes in front of the ankle and is distributed to the skin on the medial side of the foot, as far as the ball of the great toe.

The genitofemoral nerve

The genitofemoral nerve (L1, 2) emerges from the anterior surface of psoas major. Its genital branch enters the inguinal canal through the deep ring, and runs in the spermatic cord supplying cremaster and a small area of scrotal skin. The femoral nerve branch passes down behind the inguinal ligament with the femoral artery, and pierces the femoral sheath and fascia lata to supply the skin over the femoral triangle.

The obturator nerve

The obturator nerve (L2, 3, 4) emerges from the medial border of psoas major, crosses the pelvic brim medial to the sacroiliac joint, and runs along the wall of the pelvis to the obturator foramen, through which it passes above the obturator vessels. It supplies the adductor muscles and gracilis, and skin over the medial side of the thigh. Up to 57% of the population has no cutaneous branch of the obturator nerve. For this reason blockade of this nerve can only be confirmed by motor testing.

SACRAL PLEXUS

The sacral plexus (Fig. 18.2) is formed by the lumbosacral trunk and the ventral rami of the first, second, and third sacral

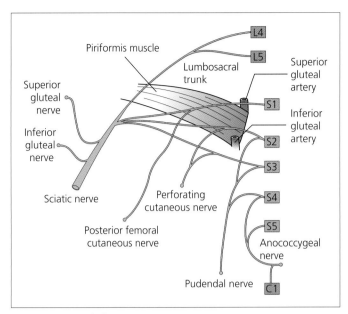

Figure 18.2 Sacral plexus anatomy.

nerves. The nerves forming the sacral plexus appear at the medial margin of the psoas major, converge toward the greater sciatic notch, and unite to form a large band located on the posterior wall of the pelvic cavity, in front of the piriformis muscle. From the anterior and posterior surfaces of the band several branches arise. The band itself is continued as the *sciatic nerve*, which splits on the back of the thigh into the *tibial and common peroneal nerves*; these two nerves sometimes arise separately in the plexus.

RELATIONS

The sacral plexus lies on the back of the pelvis between the piriformis and the pelvic fascia. In front of it are the hypogastric vessels, the ureter, and the sigmoid colon. The gluteal vessels follow the same course as the sacral nerves but in an anterior plane. The pelvic fascia is fixed medially on the anterior sacral foramina, where the sacral nerves emerge. Through this fascia, the sacral plexus lies near the rectum. Laterally, the sacral plexus lies close to the greater sciatic foramen, sandwiched by the obturator internus muscle. The sacral plexus runs in a fascial plane limited by the pelvic fascia ventrally, the piriformis dorsally, and medially and laterally by the obturator internus muscle. Hypogastric vessels are located near the sacral plexus as well as the superior gluteal artery, which passes between the lumbosacral trunk and the first sacral nerve. The inferior gluteal vessels run between the second and third sacral nerves. Collateral and terminal branches of the sacral plexus include:

- Ventral collateral branches of the sacral plexus, which are the nerve to the obturator internus muscle, the hemorrhoidal nerve, the pudendal nerve, and nerves to the various pelvic structures. All these nerves form the pudendal plexus (ventral branch of S4, anastomized with the S2 and S3 branches of the sacral plexus). These nerves supply pelvic and perineal organs.
- Dorsal collateral branches: the inferior and superior gluteal nerves, the nerves to the piriformis, gemelli, and quadratus femoris muscles.
- A single terminal branch.
- The sacral plexus, which innervates the skin of the medial part of the gluteal and posterior aspects of the thigh. It also innervates the hip joint and proximal muscles of the thigh. More caudally, the plexus extends as the sciatic nerve.

From the lower margin of the periformis, the sciatic nerve passes into the buttock on the posterior surface of the ischium. From midway between the greater trochanter and the ischial tuberosity, deep to gluteus maximus, the nerve passes vertically downward into the hamstring compartment. It lies posterior to obturator internus, gemelli, quadratus femoris, and adductor magnus, but it is crossed posteriorly by the long head of biceps femoris. The sciatic nerve usually divides into the tibial and common peroneal nerves at the upper angle of the popliteal fossa. It occasionally divides into these components within the pelvis, and the common peroneal part pierces piriformis as it leaves the pelvis.

From the apex of the popliteal fossa the tibial nerve (L4, 5, S1, 2, 3) passes vertically down deep to the heads of gastrocnemius but superficial to the popliteal vein and artery. In the popliteal fossa it supplies skin, the knee joint, calf muscles, and popliteus; it gives the sural nerve, which descends between the two heads of gastrocnemius, accompanied by the small saphenous vein to the back of the lateral malleolus and the lateral border of the foot, supplying the overlying skin. The tibial nerve passes down the leg deep to soleus, supplying the deep muscles, and reaches the medial side of the ankle, between the malleolus and the heel; here it divides into lateral and medial plantar nerves.

From the apex of the popliteal fossa, the common peroneal nerve (L4, 5, S1, 2) passes downward and laterally, medial to the biceps tendon, and turns round the neck of the fibula in the substance of peroneus longus, where it divides into superficial and deep peroneal nerves. The former supplies peroneus longus and brevis, and emerges between them to supply the skin of the lower leg and much of the dorsum of the foot. The deep peroneal nerve passes into the anterior compartment of the leg to supply the muscles here, and proceeds to the foot between the two malleoli to supply the skin of the first web space.

The sensory and motor innervation of the lower limb (Figs 18.3, 18.4) is clinically important. Knowledge of sensory

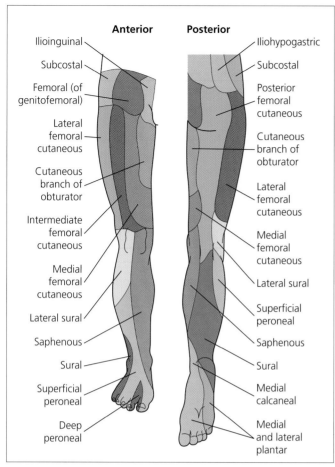

Fig. 18.3 Cutaneous innervation of the lower limb.

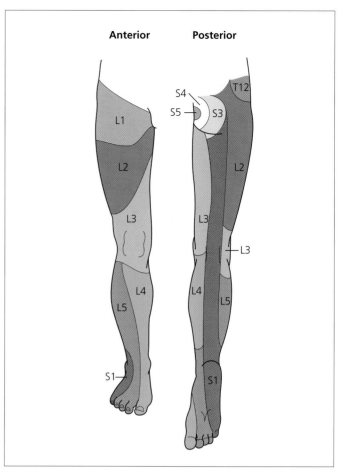

Figure 18.4 Sensory dermatomes of the lower limb.

innervation helps determine which cutaneous nerve distributions within a surgical field require blockade. Motor innervation is clinically relevant as a means of matching a peripheral nerve stimulation response to the particular nerve being stimulated.

Suggested reading

Williams PL, Warwick R, Dyson M, et al. Gray's Anatomy. 37th edn. London: Churchill Livingstone; 1989.

CHAPTER 19
Posterior sciatic block

Indications

Surgery—Surgical procedures on the lower limb from the knee distally, including Achilles tendon repair and most foot surgery (excluding the area supplied by the saphenous nerve); in combination with a lumbar plexus block for knee surgery, including total knee replacement and cruciate ligament repair.
Therapeutic—Prolonged postoperative analgesia (continuous technique); neuralgia; postamputation pain.

Contraindications

Absolute
See Chapter 4.
Relative
Hemorrhagic diathesis; anticoagulation therapy; local neural injury; patient difficulty turning into lateral decubitus position; and risk of lower extremity compartment syndrome (e.g. fresh fractures of the tibia and fibula, or especially traumatic and extensive elective orthopedic procedures of the tibia and fibula).

Anatomy

The sciatic nerve originates from the lumbar and sacral plexes and is the largest nerve in the body. The ventral rami of L4 and L5 join with those of S1, 2, and 3 to form the sciatic nerve. It is made up of two major nerves: the common peroneal and the tibial. The sciatic nerve arises on the pelvic surface of the piriformis muscle. It then passes out of the pelvis into the gluteal region through the greater sciatic foramen below the piriformis muscle, and descends between the greater trochanter of the femur and the ischial tuberosity (Figs 19.1, 19.2). Once it emerges from undercover of gluteus maximus, it becomes superficial as it passes down the posterior thigh. It divides at a variable distance, often two-thirds of the way down the posterior thigh, into the common peroneal and tibial nerves.

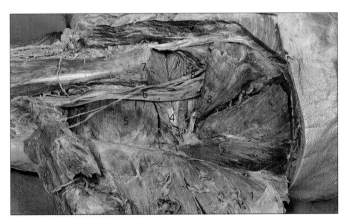

Figure 19.1 Cadaver structures illustrating anatomy pertinent to the sciatic block technique. 1, Retracted gluteus maximus; 2, gluteus medius; 3, piriformis; 4, superior and inferior gemelli; 5, quadratus femoris; 6, sciatic nerve; 7, posterior cutaneous nerve of thigh; 8, inferior gluteal nerve and artery; 9, superior gluteal artery.

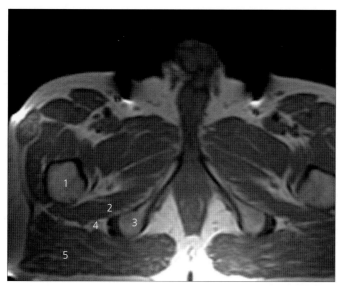

Figure 19.2 Axial T1-weighted MR image showing anatomy of sciatic nerve at site of block using the classical posterior approach of Labat. 1, Greater trochanter; 2, quadratus femoris muscle; 3, ischial tuberosity; 4, sciatic nerve; 5, gluteus maximus muscle.

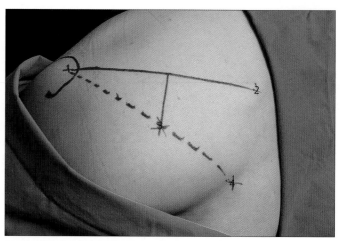

Figure 19.3 Landmarks for the posterior sciatic block. The greater trochanter (1) and posterior superior iliac spine (2) are marked. The measured distance between these points is divided equally. A perpendicular line is drawn extending into the thigh; 5 cm down this line is the needle insertion point (3). A line drawn from the greater trochanter to the sacral hiatus (4) should intersect this point.

The sciatic nerve provides sensory innervation to the posterior thigh, the lateral portion of the leg below the knee (the medial aspect being supplied by the saphenous nerve, a branch of the femoral nerve), and most of the foot. It also supplies innervation to the head of the femur and partially to the capsule of the hip joint. It supplies motor innervation to the hamstrings and all muscle groups distal to the knee.

Surface anatomy

Important bony structures for the posterior sciatic block include the greater trochanter of the femur, the posterior superior iliac spine, and the sacral hiatus. The greater trochanter can be difficult to identify exactly. It can be identified by palpating the lateral aspect of the proximal femur; 'walking' upward, one's finger tends to 'fall off' the bone when the apex of the greater trochanter is reached. The apex of the greater trochanter lies approximately a hand's breadth below the lateral aspect of the iliac crest. It is easier to palpate when the patient's hip is passively abducted to relax gluteus medius and maximus. The posterior superior iliac spine is the bony prominence at the posterior end of the iliac crest. It is directly below the 'sacral dimple' (dimple of Venus), a depression in the skin visible above the buttock, close to the midline. Palpation from the iliac crest can help to correctly identify the posterior superior iliac spine.

A consistent method of outlining the greater trochanter is needed because this is a large structure and variations can affect further marking. It is suggested that the outer perimeter of the greater trochanter is used for line drawings. A line is drawn between the posterior superior iliac spine and the greater trochanter (Fig. 19.3). This line is bisected and a perpendicular line is drawn passing downward from its midpoint. A further line is drawn from the sacral hiatus to the greater trochanter. The point at which this line intersects with the perpendicular line marks the point for needle insertion. The intersection is usually 5 cm along the perpendicular line.

Technique

As for all regional anesthetic procedures, after checking that emergency equipment is complete and in working order, intravenous access, ECG, pulse oximetry, and blood pressure monitoring are established. Asepsis is observed.

The patient is placed in the lateral decubitus (Sims) position (Fig. 19.4). A 100-mm insulated needle is used. The stimulating current is set at 0.75 mA, 2 Hz, and 0.1 ms. The needle is oriented 90° to all planes (Fig. 19.5) and advanced slowly until the appropriate muscle response is obtained: tibial nerve component produces plantar flexion and inversion of the foot, while common peroneal stimulation produces dorsiflexion and eversion of the foot. Hamstring contraction should not be accepted as a suitable response because it can be due to direct gluteal muscle stimulation.

The nerve is usually 7–9 cm deep to the skin. If bone is contacted the needle is redirected medially or laterally. The initial stimulating current should be kept at 0.75 mA or less because direct stimulation of the gluteus maximus muscle (Fig. 19.6) with higher currents can mimic sciatic nerve

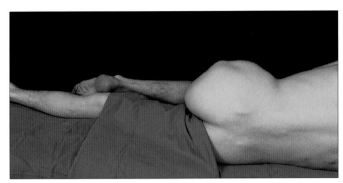

Figure 19.4 Patient position for the posterior approach to sciatic nerve block. The patient is placed in the lateral position with a slight forward tilt. The upper hip is flexed, with the foot resting on the extended knee of the lowermost limb.

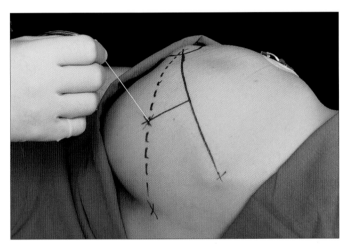

Figure 19.5 Posterior sciatic block technique. The needle is inserted in a 90° orientation to all planes.

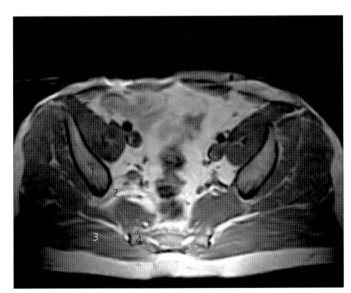

Figure 19.6 Axial T1-weighted MR image after injection of 20 mL of contrast, showing spread of contrast. Note spread toward the sacral roots and lateral wall of the pelvis. 1, Ischium; 2, sciatic nerve roots; 3, gluteus maximus muscle; 4, sacrum.

stimulation. The needle may stimulate the inferior gluteal nerve (a branch from the sacral plexus). This results in rhythmic contractions of gluteus maximus; in this circumstance the sciatic nerve is a few centimeters deeper and possibly 1 cm laterally. It is best to reattempt the block with needle insertion 1 cm lateral to the original site. The needle position is adjusted while reducing the current to 0.35 mA with maintenance of the muscle response.

Incremental injections of local anesthetic are made with repeated aspiration. For this block, 20 mL of local anesthetic is adequate.

Continuous technique

Continuous posterior sciatic block is similar to the single-shot technique, although it can be difficult to thread the catheter due to the perpendicular approach to the nerve. An alternative technique is to use the same needle insertion site but to aim the needle caudally toward the midpoint between the greater trochanter and the ischial tuberosity. An insulated Tuohy needle, oriented appropriately, may be useful to assist catheter placement with the classic posterior approach.

As with other continuous nerve block techniques, the initial dose of local anesthetic is usually injected and only then is the infusion of a more dilute local anesthetic initiated. Once the local anesthetic is injected, the catheter is carefully inserted some 5 cm beyond the tip of the needle while keeping the needle immobile. Other approaches to the sciatic nerve (including parasacral, subgluteal, and popliteal) are favored for continuous sciatic block. The catheter should be accessible with the patient supine and thus secured in a lateral direction.

◈ Adverse effects

Neural injury is rare with the use of a nerve stimulator but possible.

Local anesthetic toxicity due to intravascular injection; slow injection and careful aspiration after each 5 mL should ensure safety.

Hematoma due to puncture of inferior gluteal vessels.

Clinical Pearls

• Excellent block for Achilles tendon repair.

• Observe the foot as the needle is advanced.

• Can be used for continuous analgesia; however, there are better approaches (e.g. parasacral).

Suggested reading

di Benedetto P, Bertini L, Casati A, et al. A new posterior approach to the sciatic nerve block: a prospective, randomized comparison with the classic posterior approach. Anesth Analg 2001; 93: 1040–1044.

Labat G. Regional anesthesia: techniques and clinical applications. Philadelphia: WB Saunders; 1924.

CHAPTER 20

Anterior sciatic block

Indications

Surgery—Surgical procedures on the lower limb from the knee distally, including Achilles tendon repair and most foot surgery (excluding the area supplied by the saphenous nerve); in combination with a lumbar plexus block for knee surgery, including total knee replacement and cruciate ligament repair.
Therapeutic—Prolonged postoperative analgesia (continuous technique); neuralgia; postamputation pain.

Contraindications

Absolute
See Chapter 4.
Relative
Hemorrhagic diathesis; anticoagulation therapy; local neural injury; risk of lower extremity compartment syndrome (e.g. fresh fractures of the tibia and fibula, or especially traumatic and extensive elective orthopedic procedures of the tibia and fibula); and distorted anatomy due to fractured femur.

Anatomy

The sciatic nerve originates from the lumbar and sacral plexes and is the largest nerve in the body. The ventral rami of L4 and L5 join with those of S1, 2, and 3 to form the sciatic nerve. It is made up of two major nerves: the common peroneal and the tibial. The sciatic nerve leaves the pelvis via the sciatic foramen below piriformis, and then passes between the greater trochanter of the femur and the ischial tuberosity. It passes posterior to the lesser trochanter of the femur and here it is blocked by this approach. Once it emerges from under cover of the gluteus maximus muscle, it becomes superficial as it passes down the posterior thigh. The site of division into the common peroneal and tibial nerves is highly variable, often two-thirds the way from the gluteal region to the popliteal fossa.

The sciatic nerve provides sensory innervation to the posterior thigh, the lateral portion of the leg below the knee (the medial aspect being supplied by the saphenous nerve), and most of the foot. It also supplies sensory innervation to the head of the femur and partially to the capsule of the hip joint. It supplies motor innervation to the hamstring muscles and through its branches it supplies all muscle groups distal to the knee.

Surface anatomy

Important bony structures for the anterior sciatic block include the anterior superior iliac spine, the pubic tubercle, and the greater trochanter of the femur (Fig. 20.1). A line is drawn between the anterior superior iliac spine and the pubic tubercle (along the inguinal ligament). This line is divided into equal thirds. At the junction between the medial one-third and the lateral two-thirds, a perpendicular line is drawn extending into the thigh. A further line is drawn from the greater

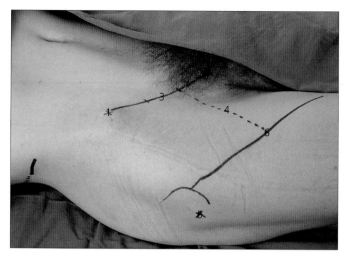

Figure 20.1 Landmarks for the anterior sciatic block. The anterior superior iliac spine and pubic tubercle are marked. The measured distance between these points is divided into equal thirds. At the junction between the medial one-third and lateral two-thirds, a perpendicular line is drawn extending into the thigh. A second horizontal line is drawn, parallel to the inguinal ligament from the greater trochanter. Where this line intersects with the vertical line is the needle insertion point. 1, Anterior superior iliac spine; 2, pubic tubercle; 3, inguinal ligament divided into equal thirds; 4, vertical line; 5, greater trochanter; 6, needle insertion point.

trochanter, parallel to the inguinal ligament. Where the perpendicular line crosses this line is the needle insertion point. Rotation of the hip due to leg position or pathology can change anatomic relations; this must be remembered when the needle insertion point is chosen. Important anatomic details include the close proximity of the femoral nerve at the site of needle insertion.

⬥ Technique

As for all regional anesthetic procedures, after checking that emergency equipment is complete and functional, intravenous access, ECG, pulse oximetry, and blood pressure monitoring are established. Asepsis is observed.

The patient is placed in the supine position with the leg in the neutral position. The operator stands on the side to be blocked, at the level of the patient's thigh. The area of the needle track is anesthetized with local anesthetic. Analgesia or sedation is very desirable for this block. A 150-mm insulated needle is inserted perpendicularly with some lateral angulation in line with the lesser trochanter of the femur (Fig. 20.2). The stimulating current is set at 1.2 mA, 2 Hz, and 0.1 ms.

On contact with the lesser trochanter the needle is withdrawn, angulated in a less lateral orientation, and advanced; the sciatic nerve is usually stimulated 3–4 cm deeper (Fig. 20.3). Total needle depth to the sciatic nerve is approximately 70% of thigh thickness; usually 8–12 cm. The needle is

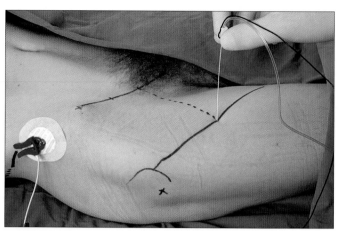

Figure 20.2 Anterior sciatic block technique. The needle is inserted with a slightly lateral orientation. If the lesser trochanter is contacted the needle is withdrawn and aimed more medially. The sciatic nerve is usually contacted at 8–12 cm from the skin, depending on thigh thickness.

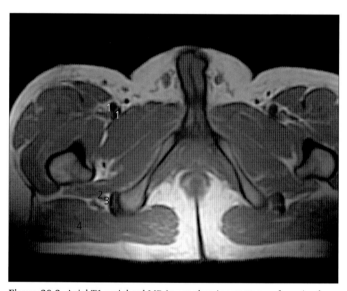

Figure 20.3 Axial T1-weighted MR image showing anatomy of proximal thigh at site of injection for anterior approach to sciatic nerve block. Note proximity of femoral nerve and vessels to track of needle. 1, Femoral nerve and vessels; 2, sciatic nerve; 3, gluteal vessels; 4, gluteus maximus.

advanced slowly until the appropriate muscle response is obtained: tibial nerve component produces plantar flexion and inversion of the foot, while common peroneal stimulation produces dorsiflexion and eversion of the foot. The needle position is adjusted while reducing the current to 0.35 mA with maintenance of the muscle response. Hamstring contraction response is not accepted. On its path to the sciatic nerve, femoral nerve stimulation may be initially found. To ensure safe practice the femoral nerve should not be blocked before sciatic nerve block.

Incremental injection of 20–30 mL of local anesthetic is made with repeated aspiration.

Continuous technique

Continuous anterior sciatic block is similar to the single-shot technique. As this approach is perpendicular to the nerve, an insulated Tuohy needle oriented appropriately may be useful to assist catheter placement.

As with other continuous nerve block techniques, the initial dose of local anesthetic is usually injected and only then is the infusion of a more dilute local anesthetic initiated. Once the local anesthetic is injected, the catheter is carefully inserted some 5 cm beyond the tip of the needle while keeping the needle immobile. Other approaches to the sciatic nerve (including parasacral, subgluteal, and popliteal) are favored for continuous sciatic block.

◈ Adverse effects

Hematoma is possible, especially if the patient is receiving anticoagulants.

Neural injury to sciatic nerve and possibly femoral nerve, especially if the femoral nerve is blocked initially.

Clinical Pearls

- This block is useful if patients cannot turn on their side.
- Fracture of the femur distorts the anatomy significantly.
- Sedation is appropriate.
- This block does not always block the posterior cutaneous nerve of thigh, which is required if a thigh tourniquet is to be used.

Suggested reading

Beck GP. Anterior approach to the sciatic nerve. Anesthesiology 1963; 24: 222–224.

CHAPTER 21
Femoral block

Indications

Surgical—Muscle biopsy; skin-graft donor site; patellar fracture fixation or wiring; combined with other techniques for saphenofemoral vein ligation; hip fracture repair and hip and knee replacement; above- and below-knee amputation; knee arthroscopy; repair of fractured shaft of femur; ankle and foot surgery.

Therapeutic—Postoperative analgesia (continuous technique) and rehabilitation in cruciate ligament reconstruction and knee replacement; postherpetic neuralgia; complex regional pain syndrome; postamputation pain; tumor-related pain.

Contraindications

Absolute
See Chapter 4.

Relative
Hemorrhagic diathesis; anticoagulation treatment; local neural injury; situations where a dense sensory block could mask the onset of lower extremity compartment syndrome (e.g. fresh fractures of the tibia and fibula, or especially traumatic and extensive elective orthopedic procedures of the tibia and fibula); and distorted anatomy due to previous surgery or trauma (e.g. prosthetic femoral artery graft).

Anatomy

The femoral nerve arises from the ventral rami of the second, third, and fourth lumbar nerves. It descends through the substance of the psoas major, emerging from the muscle at the lower part of its lateral border, and passes down between it and the iliacus muscle, deep to fascia iliacus (Fig. 21.1). It then passes behind the inguinal ligament to enter the thigh. The nerve lies deep to the fascia lata and fascia iliacus. The fascia iliacus separates it from the vascular bundle containing the femoral artery and vein (Fig. 21.2). It divides into two major branches (anterior and posterior) early in the proximal anterior thigh (Fig. 21.1).

The anterior branch provides cutaneous innervation to the skin overlying the anterior surface of the thigh and provides motor innervation to the sartorius muscle. The posterior branch provides innervation to the quadriceps muscle and the knee joint and gives rise to the saphenous nerve, which innervates the medial side of the leg below the knee.

Surface anatomy

The main landmarks for femoral nerve block are the anterior superior iliac spine, the pubic tubercle, inguinal ligament, inguinal crease, and femoral artery (Fig. 21.3). The pubic tubercle can be palpated three fingers' breadth from the midline, along the upper border of the pubis. The inguinal ligament is outlined by a line connecting the anterior superior iliac spine and the pubic tubercle.

The femoral artery lies approximately at the intersection of the medial third and lateral two-thirds of the inguinal ligament (the midinguinal point). The femoral nerve is found lateral to the femoral artery (*NAVL*: nerve, artery, vein, and ligament as you go toward the midline). The inguinal crease is a skin fold

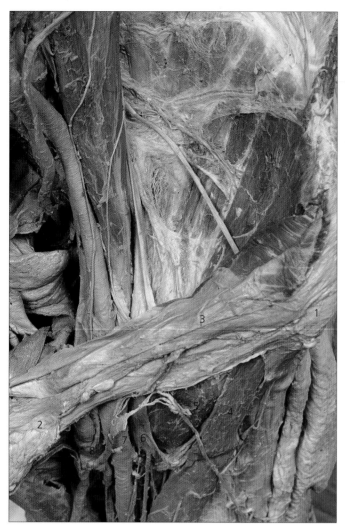

Figure 21.1 Cadaver structures illustrating anatomy relevant to femoral nerve block technique. 1, Anterior superior iliac spine; 2, pubic tubercle; 3, inguinal ligament with sectioned abdominal muscles; 4, sartorius muscle; 5, iliopsoas muscle; 6, femoral nerve; 7, femoral artery; 8, femoral vein.

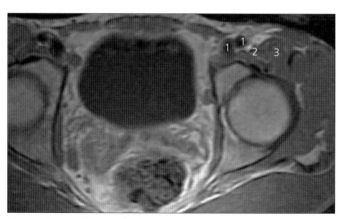

Figure 21.2 Axial T1-weighted MR image of anatomy relevant to femoral nerve block. 1, Femoral vein and artery; 2, femoral nerve; 3, iliopsoas muscle.

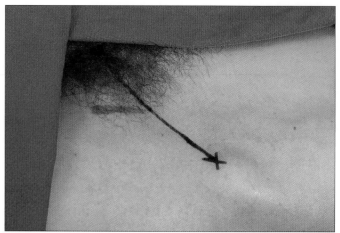

Figure 21.3 Landmarks for the femoral nerve block. The anterior superior iliac spine, pubic tubercle, and inguinal ligament are outlined. The femoral artery is identified at the level of the inguinal crease.

3–6 cm below and parallel to the inguinal ligament. Here the artery lies at its most superficial and where relations are usually constant. Below this point, the nerve begins to disappear behind the artery.

Technique

As for all regional anesthetic procedures, after checking that emergency equipment is complete and in working order, intravenous access, ECG, pulse oximetry, and blood pressure monitoring are established. Asepsis is observed.

The patient is placed in the supine position with the operator standing on the side to be blocked, at the level of the patient's thigh. The needle insertion point is infiltrated with local anesthetic using a 25-G needle. A 50-mm 23-G insulated needle is oriented in a 45° cephalad and posterior orientation lateral to the palpated femoral artery at the inguinal crease (Fig. 21.4). The stimulating current is set at 1.0 mA, 2 Hz, and 0.1 ms.

The needle is advanced slowly until the appropriate muscle response is obtained: quadriceps contraction with resultant rhythmic patellar movement. The needle position is adjusted while decreasing the current to 0.35 mA with maintenance of the muscle response. Initial stimulation currents should be less than 1.0 mA if the patient has a fractured shaft of femur, as muscle twitches can be painful. Frequently a 'pop' can be felt as the needle penetrates the fascia (usually at 2–3 cm), although this is often less obvious in elderly patients.

Incremental injections of local anesthetic are made with repeated aspiration. Fifteen milliliters of local anesthetic will adequately block the femoral nerve, but if a three-in-one block is required then use 30 mL in an adult (Figs 21.5, 21.6).

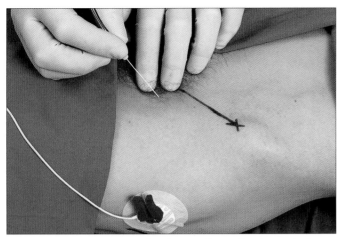

Figure 21.4 Femoral nerve block technique. The needle is inserted adjacent to the femoral artery at the level of the inguinal crease. The needle is oriented in a 45° cephalad orientation.

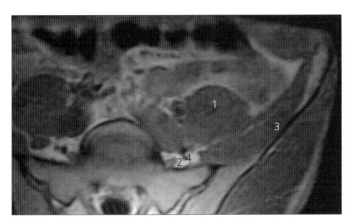

Figure 21.5 Axial T1-weighted MR image showing the spread of contrast to the obturator nerve and vessels inferomedial to the psoas muscle. This perhaps would account for the three-in-one block that can occur with this technique. It appears that the contrast spreads in a fascial plane between the psoas and iliacus muscles and 'spills over' the psoas on to its inferomedial border where the obturator nerves runs. 1, Psoas muscle; 2, contrast; 3, iliacus muscle; 4, obturator nerve.

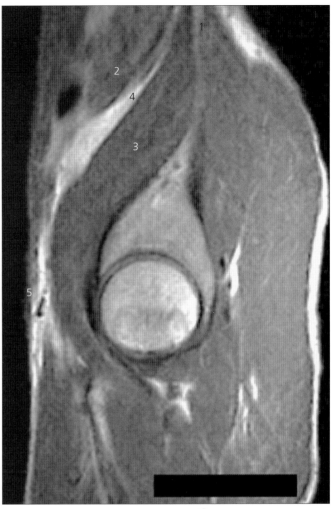

Figure 21.6 Sagittal T1-weighted MR image of spread after injection of 30 mL of contrast. Note similarity of spread in Fig. 23.3. Note that contrast covers femoral nerve and spreads laterally toward the anterior superior iliac spine, where the lateral cutaneous nerve of thigh lies. The contrast did not reach the roots of the lumbar plexus. 1, Anterior superior iliac spine; 2, psoas muscle; 3, iliacus muscle; 4, contrast spread; 5, injection site.

If a quadriceps contraction is not elicited, the needle is aimed 10° laterally. Contraction of the sartorius muscle is not appropriate; the needle should be oriented 10° laterally from this point and inserted slightly deeper. Multi-injection techniques have been described.

◈ Continuous technique

Continuous femoral block is similar to the single-shot technique. The insertion point, however, is slightly above the inguinal crease to avoid the skin breaking at the femoral crease.

As with other continuous nerve block techniques, the initial dose of local anesthetic is usually injected and only then is the infusion of a more dilute local anesthetic initiated. Once the local anesthetic is injected, the catheter is carefully inserted some 5 cm beyond the tip of the needle while keeping the needle immobile. When the catheter meets resistance at the tip of the needle, the needle may be repositioned at a different angle or rotated to facilitate advancement of the catheter. Once the catheter is inserted, the needle is withdrawn while simultaneously advancing the catheter to prevent its dislodgment. The catheter is secured with a transparent dressing.

Adverse effects

Hematoma is unusual, even if the artery is perforated; pressure should be applied to the needle insertion site.

Neural injuries are extremely rare.

Local anesthetic toxicity due to injection into the femoral artery; slow injection and careful aspiration after each 5 mL should ensure safety.

Clinical Pearls

• Femoral block is more difficult to perform in patients with a fractured femur, because the anatomy is frequently altered due to hematoma formation and external rotation of the lower limb.

• The three-in-one block is similar to the classical femoral nerve block; larger volumes of local anesthetic and distal digital pressure are technique modifications. Obturator anesthesia tends to be less reliable with the three-in-one than with the lumbar plexus approach. Lateral cutaneous nerve of thigh anesthesia tends to be less reliable with the three-in-one than with the iliacus compartment block.

• Femoral block is a superficial block and does not result in significant patient discomfort; thus light premedication usually suffices.

Saphenous block

The saphenous nerve is a branch of the femoral nerve and provides cutaneous sensation to the medial aspect of the ankle and a variable portion of the medial foot. It is probably most consistently blocked by femoral block; however, it can be blocked separately at the level of the knee.

The saphenous nerve passes within the adductor canal beneath the sartorius muscle, and then curves around the

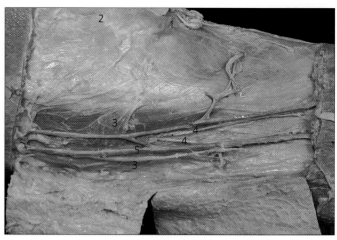

Figure 21.7 Cadaver structures illustrating anatomy relevant to saphenous nerve block at the knee. 1, Tibial tuberosity; 2, patella; 3, semitendinosus and semimembranosus muscles; 4, saphenous nerve branches; 5, long saphenous vein.

posteriomedial aspect of the knee to divide into branches along the anteriomedial aspect of the proximal tibia (Fig. 21.7).

Several techniques for block of the saphenous nerve have been described. The tibial tuberosity can be felt as a bony prominence inferior to the patella. The gastrocnemius muscle can be palpated medially from the tibial tuberosity and is a relevant anatomic landmark for saphenous nerve block. The saphenous nerve is blocked by subcutaneous injection from the tibial tuberosity to the gastrocnemius muscle. An ellipse of local anesthetic is injected with 4–6 mL of solution.

Suggested reading

Casati A, Fanelli G, Beccaria P, et al. The effects of the single or multiple injection technique on the onset time of femoral nerve blocks with 0.75% ropivacaine. Anesth Analg 2000; 91: 181–184.

Marhofer P, Nasel C, Sitzwohl C, et al. Magnetic resonance imaging of the distribution of local anesthetic during the three-in-one block. Anesth Analg 2000; 90: 119–124.

Vloka JD, Hadzic A, Drobnik L, et al. Anatomical landmarks for femoral nerve block: a comparison of four needle insertion sites. Anesth Analg 1999; 89: 1467–1470.

Winnie AP, Ramamurthy S, Durrani Z. The inguinal paravascular technique of lumbar plexus anesthesia: the '3-in-1 block'. Anesth Analg 1973; 52: 989–996.

CHAPTER 22
Psoas block

◈ Indications

Surgical—Surgical procedures on the upper leg; combined with a sciatic nerve block when necessary; skin grafting from anterior, lateral, and medial thigh; surgery on the anterior knee and patella.

Therapeutic—Prolonged postoperative analgesia (continuous technique); amputation pain; postherpetic neuralgia; low back pain.

◈ Contraindications

Absolute
See Chapter 4.
Relative
Bleeding diathesis; anticoagulation therapy; lumbar scoliosis; and local neural injury.

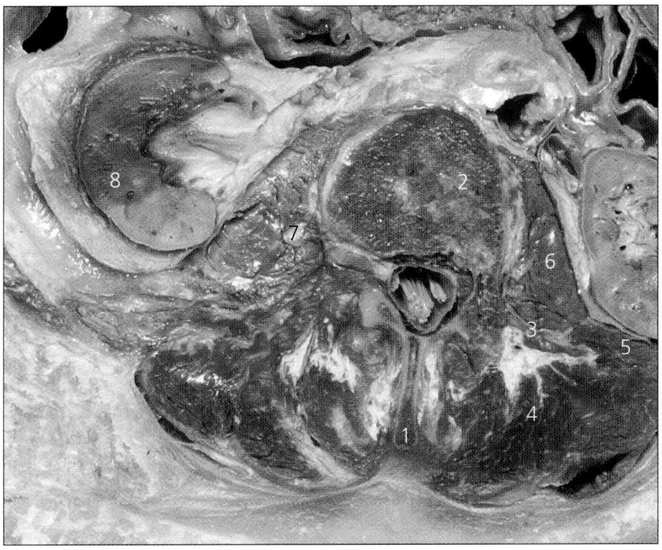

Figure 22.1 Lumbar (L2) sagittal section illustrating anatomy relevant to the psoas block.1, Spinous process; 2, vertebral body; 3, transverse process; 4, erector spinae muscle; 5, quadratus lumborum muscle; 6, psoas muscle; 7, lumbar nerve; 8, kidney.

◈ Anatomy

The lumbar plexus is formed by the ventral rami of the first three lumbar nerves and the greater part of the ventral ramus of the fourth. It lies in front of the transverse processes of the lumbar vertebrae, deep within the psoas major muscle (Fig. 22.1). The nerve roots of the lumbar plexus lie in a 'cleavable' space in the psoas major muscle (Fig. 22.2). The space is limited superiorly by the insertion of psoas major on the body of the vertebrae; posteriorly by the lumbar transverse processes and peridural space; and anteriorly by the aponeurotic continuation of the fascia iliaca.

Anatomically, psoas muscle is regarded as one mass and there is no 'compartment' as such within the muscle. Nevertheless, injectate does infiltrate the muscle (Fig. 22.3) and covers the lumbar roots and nerves running within the muscle.

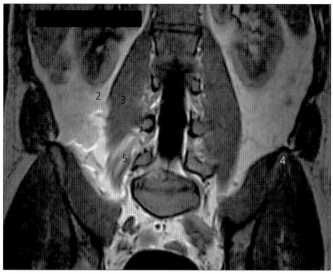

Figure 22.2 Coronal T1-weighted MR image of anatomy relevant to psoas block. 1, Right kidney; 2, retroperitoneal space; 3, psoas muscle; 4, anterior superior iliac spine; 5, lumbar nerve roots; 6, iliacus muscle.

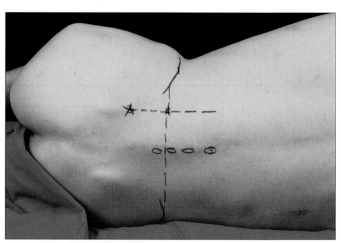

Figure 22.4 Landmarks for the psoas block. The iliac crest and posterior superior iliac spine are marked. A line is drawn joining both iliac crests. A line is drawn, parallel to the spine, which passes through the posterior superior iliac spine. Where both lines intersect is the needle insertion point. 1, Iliac crest; 2, posterior superior iliac spine; 3, spinous processes; 4, needle insertion point.

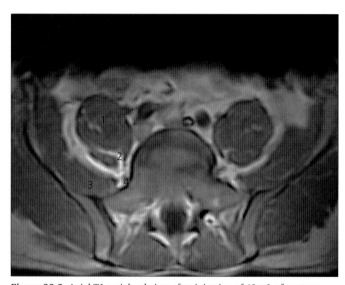

Figure 22.3 Axial T1-weighted view after injection of 40 mL of contrast. Note spread *through* the psoas muscle. This demonstrates well the cleavable nature of the psoas muscle. 1, Psoas muscle; 2, potential space created by contrast spread; 3, iliacus muscle; 4, obturator nerve.

The roots join and form the lumbar plexus within the psoas muscle. Branches of the plexus include femoral, obturator, and lateral cutaneous nerve of thigh.

Surface anatomy

Important landmarks for the psoas block include the iliac crests, the posterior superior iliac spine, and the vertebral column (Fig. 22.4). The posterior superior iliac spine is the bony prominence at the posterior end of the iliac crest. It is directly below the 'sacral dimple' (dimple of Venus), a dimple in the skin visible above the buttock, close to the midline.

A vertical line is drawn between the highest points of the iliac crests. This is called the Tuffier line and passes through the disc space of L3 and L4. A second line is drawn parallel to the spinous processes and passes through the posterior superior iliac spine on the side to be blocked. Where these two lines intersect is the needle insertion point (usually 4–5 cm from the midline).

Technique

As for all regional anesthetic procedures, after checking that emergency equipment is complete and functional, intravenous access, ECG, pulse oximetry, and blood pressure monitoring are established. Asepsis is observed.

The lumbar plexus can be blocked with a single injection as it passes through the psoas muscle. As this is a deep block, sedation is indicated for patient comfort and the needle track should be anesthetized with local anesthetic. The patient is placed in the lateral position with the side to be blocked uppermost and the hips flexed (Fig. 22.5). This block is commonly performed combined with a sciatic nerve block. The two blocks can be performed with the patient in the same position if the classical Labat posterior approach is used.

A 100-mm insulated stimulating needle is used. The stimulating current is set at 1.0 mA, 2 Hz, and 0.1 ms. The needle is inserted perpendicular to the skin (Fig. 22.6) and

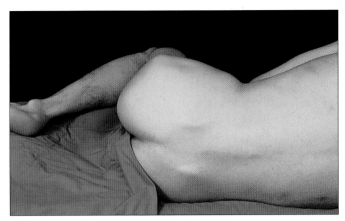

Figure 22.5 Patient position for the psoas block. The patient is placed in the lateral position with both hips flexed.

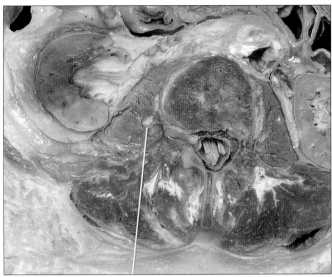

Figure 22.7 Lumbar (L2) sagittal section illustrating needle orientation and endpoint for the psoas block.

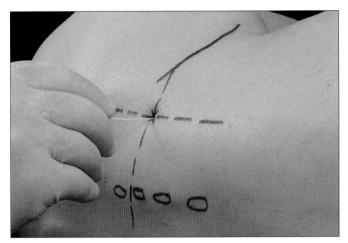

Figure 22.6 Psoas block technique. The needle is oriented perpendicular to the skin.

transverses the following structures: skin, fat, erector spinae, and quadratus lumborum muscles (Fig. 22.7). Contact with the transverse process is an important reference point. The plexus lies 2–3 cm deep to the transverse process, 7–9 cm from the skin. If the transverse process (L4) is contacted, the needle should be redirected below because passing above increases the risk of renal puncture. Normal kidney extends down to L3 level.

Correct needle position is indicated by quadriceps muscle contraction. After eliciting the appropriate muscle contraction, the current is then reduced to 0.35 mA while maintaining the response. Hip flexion (direct muscle stimulation of psoas major) indicates a needle position that is too deep; intraperitoneal, aortic, or caval puncture also indicate too deep a position. Adductor muscle contraction or venous puncture (ascending lumbar vein) indicates a too medial orientation. Medial puncture should also be avoided to reduce risk of intrathecal or epidural injection. Stimulation of the sciatic

nerve indicates needle puncture that is too caudad. Renal puncture indicates needle insertion that is too lateral and too cephalad.

When the needle position is satisfactory, incremental injection of local anesthetic is made with repeated aspiration for blood and cerebrospinal fluid.

A modification of this approach has been described by Capdevila et al.

Continuous technique

The approach described above is suitable for continuous techniques. Continuous psoas block is similar to the single-shot technique. As this approach is perpendicular to the plexus, an insulated Tuohy needle, oriented appropriately, may be useful to assist catheter placement. However, it is possible using an uninsulated Tuohy needle and a loss of resistance technique.

As with other continuous nerve block techniques, the initial dose of local anesthetic is usually injected and only then is the infusion of a more dilute local anesthetic initiated. Once the local anesthetic is injected, the catheter is carefully inserted some 5 cm beyond the tip of the needle while keeping the needle immobile. As there is a risk of epidural spread with the psoas block, large volumes of local anesthetic should be injected slowly, with appropriate patient observation.

Continuous lumbar plexus block is a safe alternative to continuous epidural analgesia, especially when anticoagulants are administered perioperatively. The catheter should be accessible with the patient supine and thus secured in a lateral direction.

◈ Adverse effects

Hematoma: the aorta, vena cava, or lumbar vessels can be punctured.

Spinal or epidural anesthesia due to intrathecal or epidural injection; it is thus imperative to monitor these patients carefully during and after injection of local anesthetic.

Renal or ureteric injury is a particular risk with techniques above L4.

Neural injury is rare.

Local anesthetic toxicity is possible due to the multiplicity of vessels in the area.

Clinical Pearls

• Quadriceps contraction on stimulation is an excellent indicator of correct needle position.

• Combined with sciatic nerve block, this block gives excellent anesthesia of the leg and is especially useful for knee surgery.

• For hip surgery, the T12 nerve needs to be anesthetized separately.

• Suitable for continuous techniques for prolonged pain relief in hip and knee surgery.

Suggested reading

Chayen D, Nathan H, Chayen M. The psoas compartment block. Anesthesiology 1976; 45: 95–99.

Capdevila X, Macaire P, Dodure C et al. Continuous psoas compartment block for postoperative analgesia after total hip arthroplasty: new landmarks, technical guidelines, and clinical evaluation. Anesth. Analg 2002; 94: 1606–1613.

CHAPTER 23

Iliacus block

Indications

Surgical—Muscle biopsy; skin-graft donor site; patellar fracture fixation or wiring; combined with other techniques for saphenofemoral vein ligation; hip fracture repair and hip and knee replacement; above- and below-knee amputation; knee arthroscopy; repair of fractured shaft of femur; ankle and foot surgery.

Therapeutic—Postoperative analgesia (continuous technique) and rehabilitation in cruciate ligament reconstruction and knee replacement; postherpetic neuralgia; complex regional pain syndrome; postamputation pain; tumor-related pain.

Contraindications

Absolute
See Chapter 4.
Relative
Hemorrhagic diathesis; anticoagulation treatment; local neural injury; and risk of lower extremity compartment syndrome (e.g. fresh fractures of the tibia and fibula, or especially traumatic and extensive elective orthopedic procedures of the tibia and fibula).

Anatomy

The iliacus fascia covers the iliacus and psoas muscles in the pelvis and descends into the thigh with these muscles (Fig. 23.1). The femoral nerve lies anterior to the psoas muscle initially, with the lateral cutaneous nerve of thigh lateral to the psoas muscle and obturator nerve medial. At the inguinal ligament the femoral nerve lies in a gutter between the psoas and iliacus muscles. These nerves thus lie beneath the iliacus fascia (Fig. 23.1). Spread of local anesthetic (Figs 23.2, 23.3) beneath the iliacus fascia produces a higher success rate of anesthesia of the femoral nerve, lateral cutaneous nerve of thigh, and obturator nerves than the femoral nerve block technique.

Surface anatomy

The main landmarks for iliacus block are the anterior superior iliac spine, pubic tubercle, and inguinal ligament. The pubic tubercle can be palpated three fingers' breadth from the midline, along the upper border of the pubis.

The inguinal ligament is outlined by a line connecting the anterior superior iliac spine and the pubic tubercle. The inguinal ligament is divided into equal thirds. At the junction between the outer one-third and inner two-thirds, a perpendicular line is drawn; 1 cm along this line is the needle insertion point (Fig. 23.4). The femoral artery can be palpated 2–3 cm more medially in the groin.

It is important to remember that with a fractured neck of femur these relations may change.

Technique

As for all regional anesthetic procedures, after checking that emergency equipment is complete and in working order,

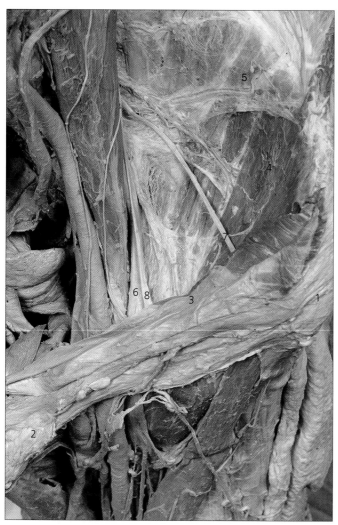

Figure 23.1 Cadaver structures illustrating anatomy relevant to the iliacus block technique. 1, Anterior superior iliac spine; 2, pubic tubercle; 3, inguinal ligament with abdominal muscles sectioned and removed; 4, iliacus muscle; 5, iliacus fascia; 6, femoral nerve; 7, lateral cutaneous nerve of thigh; 8, genitofemoral nerve. The obturator nerve is not visible on medial aspect of psoas muscle.

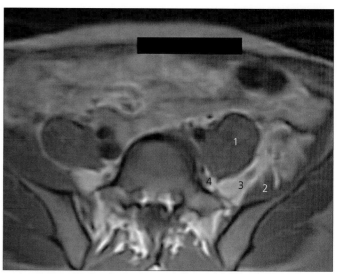

Figure 23.2 Axial T1-weighted MR image after injection of 40 mL of contrast, showing spread of injectate. Compare with Fig. 21.5. Note contrast surrounding femoral and obturator nerves. Spread is via the plane between the iliacus and psoas muscles. 1, Psoas muscle; 2, iliacus muscle; 3, femoral nerve; 4, obturator nerve.

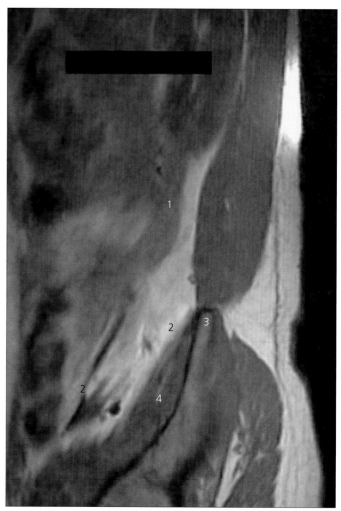

Figure 23.3 (Right) Sagittal T1-weighted MR image demonstrating spread of contrast toward anterior superior iliac spine, where the lateral cutaneous nerve of thigh lies. Compare with Fig. 21.6. 1, Psoas muscle; 2, contrast spread; 3, anterior superior iliac spine; 4, iliacus muscle.

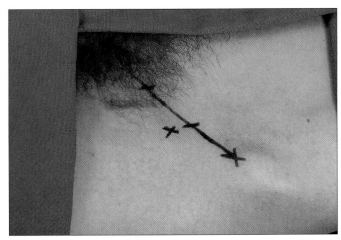

Figure 23.4 Landmarks for the iliacus block. The anterior superior iliac spine, pubic tubercle, and inguinal ligament are outlined. The inguinal ligament is divided into equal thirds. At the junction between the outer one-third and inner two-thirds, a perpendicular line is drawn extending into the thigh; 1 cm down this line is the needle insertion point.

intravenous access, ECG, pulse oximetry, and blood pressure monitoring are established. Asepsis is observed.

The patient is placed in the supine position with the operator standing on the side to be blocked, at the level of the patient's thigh. Having outlined landmarks, the needle insertion point is infiltrated with local anesthetic using a 25-G needle. An 18-G Tuohy needle is inserted perpendicular to the skin (Fig. 23.5). An initial loss of resistance is identified on penetrating the fascia lata. A second loss of resistance indicates penetration of the fascia iliaca. No muscle response is sought. Incremental injection of local anesthetic (30–40 mL) is made

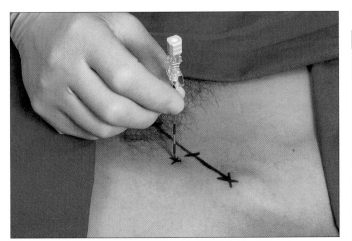

Figure 23.5 Iliacus block technique. The epidural needle is inserted perpendicular to the skin. A loss of resistance technique is used to identify the iliacus fascia.

with repeated aspiration. No resistance to injection should be present.

As this is a compartment block, volume of local anesthetic is important. The compartment is highly vascular, suggesting that inclusion of vasoconstrictor agents, such as adrenaline (epinephrine) and clonidine, with local anesthetic may be useful.

Continuous technique

Continuous iliacus block is similar to the single-shot technique. The needle bevel should be directed in a cephalad direction. As with other continuous nerve block techniques, the initial dose of local anesthetic is usually injected and only then is the infusion of a more dilute local anesthetic initiated. Once the local anesthetic is injected, the catheter is carefully inserted some 5 cm beyond the tip of the needle while keeping the needle immobile. Once the catheter is inserted, the needle is withdrawn while simultaneously advancing the catheter to prevent its dislodgment. The catheter is secured with a transparent dressing.

Adverse effects

Hematoma: note that needle insertion is more lateral than with the femoral nerve block technique, which decreases the risk of intravascular injection.

Neural injuries are extremely rare; the technique is easy to perform on an awake patient, which increases safety.

Local anesthetic toxicity due to overdosage or intravascular diffusion can cause symptoms of CNS toxicity. Slow injection of local anesthetics and repeated aspiration decrease the incidence of this complication.

Clinical Pearls

- The alteration in tissue resistance is often better appreciated by advancing a blunt needle (e.g. a Tuohy needle), held like a pen, with small side-to-side or vertical oscillations.

- The distance from the femoral artery provides this margin of safety.

- Asking the patient to cough increases intra-abdominal pressure and results in forced expulsion of local anesthetic through a needle placed beneath the iliacus fascia.

Suggested reading

Capdevila X, Biboulet P, Bouregba M, et al. Comparison of the three-in-one and fascia iliaca compartment blocks in adults: clinical and radiographic analysis. Anesth Analg 1998; 86: 1039–1044.

Kizelshteyn G, Crevecoeur E. Anatomic consideration of the fascia iliaca compartment block. Anesth Analg 1990; 71: 210–212.

Paut O, Sallabery M, Schreiber-Deturmeny E, et al. Continuous fascia iliaca compartment block in children: a prospective evaluation of plasma bupivacaine concentrations, pain scores, and side effects. Anesth Analg 2001; 92: 1159–1163.

CHAPTER 24
Lateral cutaneous nerve of thigh block

Indications

Surgical—Surgical procedures involving the lateral side of thigh and knee, including skin-graft harvesting from the lateral thigh, or removal of skin lesions from the lateral thigh. *Therapeutic*—Neuralgia; differential diagnosis of thigh pain; postoperative pain relief.

Contraindications

Absolute
See Chapter 4.
Relative
Bleeding diathesis; anticoagulation therapy; and obesity making palpation of the anterior superior iliac spine difficult.

Anatomy

The lateral cutaneous nerve of the thigh (L2, 3) is a purely sensory nerve. It emerges from the psoas muscle along its lateral border. It runs deep to the iliac fascia on the iliacus muscle, emerging immediately inferior and medial to the anterior superior iliac spine. After crossing under the inguinal ligament, it passes through the origin of the sartorius muscle and travels beneath the fascia lata, before dividing into a large descending branch and a smaller posterior branch, a variable distance below the inguinal ligament (Fig. 24.1). The branches

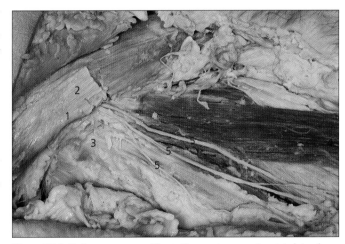

Figure 24.1 Cadaver structures illustrating anatomy pertinent to lateral cutaneous nerve of thigh block technique. 1, Anterior superior iliac spine; 2, inguinal ligament; 3, fascia lata; 4, sartorius muscle; 5, divisions of the lateral cutaneous nerve of thigh.

pierce the fascia lata separately. The descending branch innervates the anterolateral thigh as far as the knee; the posterior branch innervates the lateral aspect of the thigh to midthigh level.

Surface anatomy

Important anatomic landmarks for block of the lateral cutaneous nerve of thigh include the anterior superior iliac

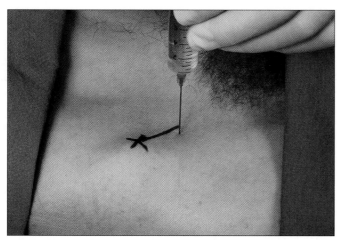

Figure 24.2 Lateral cutaneous nerve of thigh block technique. The needle insertion point is 2 cm medial and 2 cm inferior from the anterior superior iliac spine (below the inguinal ligament). The needle is inserted perpendicular to the skin.

spine and the inguinal ligament. The needle insertion site is located 2 cm medial and 2 cm inferior to the anterior superior iliac spine (Fig. 24.2). This should be below the inguinal ligament, unlike the needle insertion site for the ilioinguinal nerve block.

Technique

As for all regional anesthetic procedures, after checking that emergency equipment is complete and functional, intravenous access, ECG, pulse oximetry, and blood pressure monitoring are established. Asepsis is observed.

The patient is placed in the supine position. A 30-mm 23-G hypodermic needle is inserted perpendicular to the skin. The needle is advanced in a controlled, intermittent fashion. Penetration of the fascia lata is indicated by a 'pop'. Injection is performed above and below the fascia lata, in a medial to lateral direction. For this block, 10 mL of local anesthetic is adequate.

Adverse effects

Hematoma can occur.

Unwanted anesthesia due to spread of local anesthetic to femoral, ilioinguinal, or iliohypogastric nerves can occur if larger than necessary volumes of local anesthetic are used.

Suggested reading

Brown TCK, Dickens DRV. A new approach to lateral cutaneous nerve of thigh block. Anaesth Intensive Care 1986; 14: 126–127.

Hopkins PM, Ellis FR, Halsall PJ. Evaluation of local anesthetic blockade of the lateral femoral cutaneous nerve. Anesthesia 1991; 46: 95–96.

CHAPTER 25

Popliteal block

◈ Indications

Surgical—Foot surgery; below-knee amputations; Achilles tendon surgery; in conjunction with a femoral or saphenous block for short saphenous vein surgery and fixation of ankle fractures.

Therapeutic—Mobilization of the ankle; complex regional pain syndrome; postamputation pain; tumor-related pain.

◈ Contraindications

Absolute

See Chapter 4.

Relative

Hemorrhagic diathesis; anticoagulation treatment; distorted anatomy (due to previous surgery or trauma); and risk of lower extremity compartment syndrome (e.g. fresh fractures of the tibia and fibula, or especially traumatic and extensive elective orthopedic procedures of the tibia and fibula).

◈ Anatomy

The popliteal fossa is defined as the space between the skin, the femur anteriorly and the biceps femoris muscle laterally, the semitendinosus and semimembranosus muscles medially, and inferiorly by both heads of gastrocnemius (Figs 25.1, 25.2). The space is mostly filled with fat and contains in its

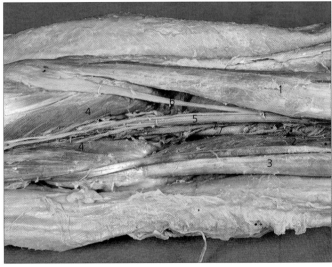

Figure 25.1 Cadaver structures illustrating anatomy relevant to the posterior popliteal block technique. 1, Biceps femoris; 2, semimembranosus; 3, semitendinosus; 4, gastrocnemius; 5, tibial nerve; 6, common peroneal nerve; 7, popliteal vessels.

anterolateral aspect the popliteal vessels and nerves. The sciatic nerve is formed from roots L4 to S2 (and occasionally S3) and consists of two distinct divisions—the tibial and common peroneal nerves—which share a common epineural sheath from their origin to the popliteal fossa. The two nerves innervate the entire leg below the knee except for the antero-medial leg and foot, which are innervated by the saphenous nerve (L2, 3, 4).

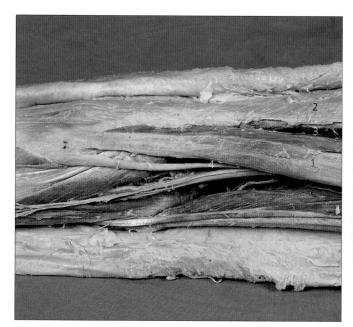

Figure 25.2 Cadaver structures illustrating anatomy relevant to the lateral popliteal block technique. 1, Biceps femoris; 2, vastus lateralis; 3, intermuscular groove; 4, common peroneal nerve.

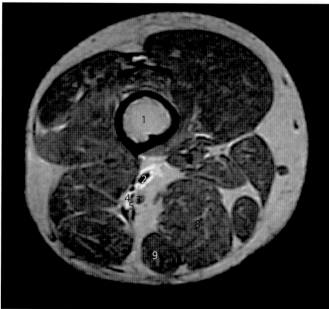

Figure 25.3 Axial T1-weighted MR image of thigh 5 cm superior to popliteal crease. Note separate tibial and common peroneal components of sciatic nerve lateral to midline. 1, Femur; 2, profunda femoris artery; 3, tibial nerve; 4, common peroneal nerve; 5, sural communicating nerve; 6, biceps femoris muscle; 7, gracilis muscle; 8, semimembranous muscle; 9, semitendinosus muscle.

The sciatic nerve branches in the region of the distal thigh (Fig. 25.3), anywhere between 4 and 13 cm above the popliteal crease, although occasionally they can run as two separate nerves from the sciatic foramen. The tibial nerve is the larger of the two branches and runs parallel and slightly lateral to the midline. Inferiorly, it passes between the heads of the gastrocnemius muscle. The common peroneal nerve runs laterally along the medial aspect of the biceps femoris muscle. After bifurcation the tibial nerve immediately gives off the sural nerve, which innervates the lateral aspect of the foot. The common peroneal nerve also gives off a sural communicating nerve (Fig. 25.4), and once it is below the head of the fibula it divides into superficial and deep peroneal nerves. The nerves lie more superficial and lateral to the popliteal vessels in the popliteal fossa and about midway between the skin and the posterior aspect of the femur, at a depth of 1.5–2 cm in adults.

◈ Surface anatomy

The main landmarks for the lateral popliteal block include the superior aspect of the patella and a muscular groove between the biceps femoris and vastus lateralis muscles (Fig. 25.5). Identification of this groove is difficult in obese patients and should be mastered prior to procedure. This is easily felt when patients flex their leg against resistance.

The main landmarks for the posterior popliteal block include skin crease of the knee joint and biceps femoris muscle

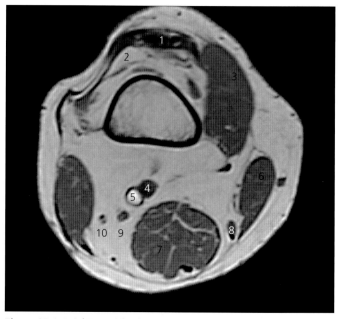

Figure 25.4 Axial T1-weighted MR image showing anatomy at the level of the superior border of the patella. Note relations of the common peroneal 10. and tibial nerves 9. to popliteal vessels. The common peroneal and tibial components are 7 mm apart in this individual. The sural communicating nerve is marked. 1, Quadriceps tendon, 2, patella; 3, vastus medialis muscle; 4, popliteal artery; 5, popliteal vein; 6, sartorius muscle; 7, semimembranosus muscle; 8, gracilis muscle.

intravenous access, ECG, pulse oximetry, and blood pressure monitoring are established. Asepsis is observed.

Lateral approach

The patient is placed supine with the lower limb in the neutral position. The feet should be extended beyond the edge of the table in order to better discern the response to nerve stimulation (Fig. 25.7). A small sandbag underneath the knee or a pillow under the thigh facilitates the technique. The upper border of the patella is identified and a line is drawn vertically downward to the patient trolley. The groove between the lateral border of vastus lateralis and the biceps femoris tendon is identified. The intersection of the two lines is the needle insertion point.

Having outlined landmarks, the needle insertion point is infiltrated with local anesthetic using a 25-G needle. A 50-mm 21-G insulated needle is inserted at 30° to the horizontal plane, ensuring that the needle is directed away from the popliteal vessels (Fig. 25.8). The stimulating current is set at 1.0 mA, 2 Hz, and 0.1 ms. The needle is advanced slowly until the appropriate muscle response is obtained. The needle position is adjusted while decreasing the current to 0.35 mA with maintenance of the muscle response.

The common peroneal and tibial nerves are identified by their muscular responses: plantar flexion or inversion of the foot for the tibial nerve, and dorsiflexion or eversion of the foot for the common peroneal nerve. With failure to elicit nerve stimulation, needle insertion is moved in an anteropostero direction within the groove.

The common peroneal nerve is usually found first because it is located more laterally (Fig. 25.9). After the first nerve is stimulated, at less than 0.5 mA, 10 mL of local anesthetic is

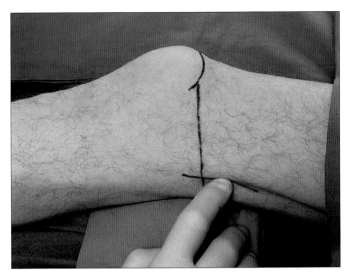

Figure 25.5 Landmarks for the lateral popliteal block. A vertical line is drawn from the superior aspect of the patella. A second line is drawn that outlines the groove between vastus lateralis and biceps femoris. Where both lines intersect is the needle insertion point.

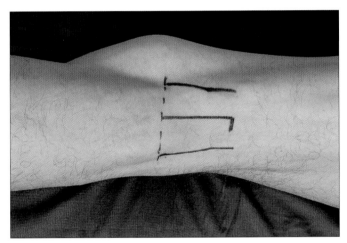

Figure 25.6 Landmarks for the posterior popliteal block. A line is drawn that outlines the knee crease. Muscular boundaries formed by semimembranosus and semitendinosus medially and biceps femoris laterally are outlined. At the midpoint of the knee crease a perpendicular line is drawn into the thigh. The needle insertion point is 5 cm along this line and 1 cm laterally.

laterally, and semimembranosus muscle medially (Fig. 25.6). The patient can be asked to flex the leg to identify the margins of the popliteal fossa. Absence of bony landmarks with the posterior approach increases the learning curve with this approach.

◈ Technique

As for all regional anesthetic procedures, after checking that emergency equipment is complete and in working order,

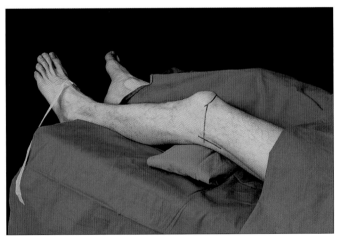

Figure 25.7 Patient position for the lateral popliteal block. The patient is placed in the supine position with the feet visible beyond the edge of the patient trolley. Note the sandbag beneath the knee and tape maintaining neutral leg position.

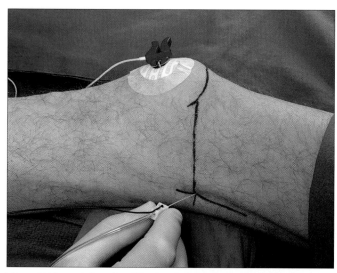

Figure 25.8 Lateral popliteal block technique. The needle is inserted at 30° to the horizontal plane.

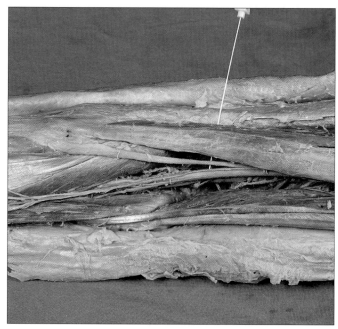

Figure 25.9 Lateral popliteal block technique. The needle passes through the intermuscular groove and is most likely to encounter the common peroneal nerve initially.

injected slowly after careful aspiration. Then the amplitude of the nerve stimulator is increased to 2 mA and the needle is advanced slightly. The tibial nerve is located approximately 1–3 cm more medially and a further 10 mL of local anesthetic is injected. With prior injection of local anesthetic, the second nerve should be found in a short time period if possible, because there is a theoretical risk of nerve damage when the surrounding area becomes anesthetized.

A muscular twitch may be elicited in the biceps femoris muscle. This is direct muscle stimulation and indicates that the needle trajectory is correct. Inversion is a muscular movement, which is common to both nerves, caused by the action of the tibialis posterior muscle innervated by the tibial nerve, and the tibialis anterior muscle innervated by the common peroneal nerve. Eliciting strong inversion results in an over 60% success rate for block of both nerves.

Continuous technique

Continuous lateral popliteal block is similar to the single-shot technique. As with other continuous nerve block techniques, the initial dose of local anesthetic is usually injected and only then is the infusion of a more dilute local anesthetic initiated. Once the local anesthetic is injected, the catheter is carefully inserted some 5 cm beyond the tip of the needle while keeping the needle immobile. When the catheter meets resistance at the tip of the needle, the needle may be repositioned at a different angle or rotated to facilitate advancement of the catheter. Once the catheter is inserted, the needle is withdrawn while simultaneously advancing the catheter to prevent its dislodgment.

Posterior approach

The patient is placed in the prone or lateral position. The feet should be extended beyond the edge of the table in order to better discern the response to nerve stimulation (Fig. 25.10). The patient is asked to flex the leg to identify the margins of the popliteal fossa. The fossa is divided into lateral and medial triangles with the crease at the base of these triangles. The site of needle insertion is 5 cm above the popliteal crease and 1 cm lateral to the midline of the triangle.

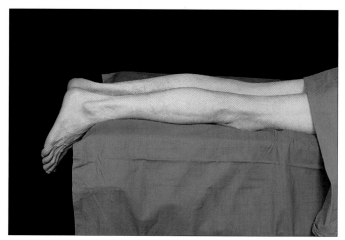

Figure 25.10 Patient position for the posterior popliteal block. The patient is placed in the prone position with the feet visible beyond the edge of the table.

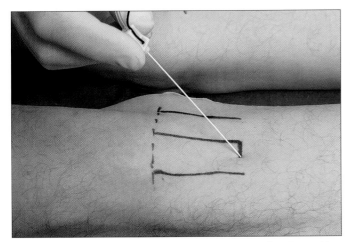

Figure 25.11 Posterior popliteal block technique. The needle is inserted in a 45° cephalad orientation.

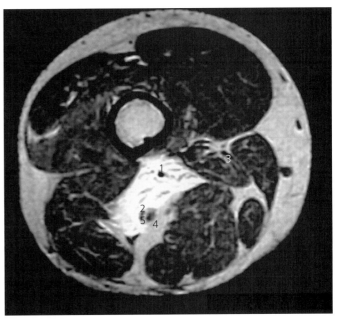

Figure 25.12 Axial T1-weighted MR image showing spread of 20 mL of contrast injected at same level as in Fig. 25.3. Stimulating needle-stimulated common peroneal component. Note the wide spread of contrast in the intermuscular plane, which is significantly widened by the volume of contrast. Note also the apparent movement of the nerves medially and also that contrast does not completely surround the tibial nerve but spreads to areas unnecessary for sciatic nerve block. 1, Profunda femoris artery; 2, femoral vessels; 3, common peroneal nerve; 4, tibial nerve; 5, sural communicating nerve.

After raising a skin wheal of local anesthetic, a 50-mm 21-G insulated needle is inserted in a 45° cephalad orientation (Fig. 25.11). The stimulating current is set at 1.0 mA, 2 Hz, and 0.1 ms. The needle is advanced slowly until the appropriate muscle response is obtained. The needle position is adjusted while decreasing the current to 0.35 mA with maintenance of the muscle response.

Usually the nerves are located at a depth of 1.5–2 cm, resulting in either plantar flexion and inversion (tibial nerve) or dorsiflexion and eversion (common peroneal nerve) of the foot. When the described responses are not obtained on the first needle pass, the needle is withdrawn and redirected slightly laterally using the same insertion site. Then 30–40 mL of local anesthetic is injected (Fig. 25.12). A single injection technique is usually sufficient with the posterior approach, because the nerves lie in close proximity.

Continuous technique

Continuous posterior popliteal block is similar to the single-shot technique.

◈ Adverse effects

Hematoma.

Neural injuries are extremely rare. When using the lateral approach, be mindful of the time taken to find the second nerve because there is a considerable amount of local anesthetic in the area after the first injection.

Local anesthetic toxicity due to intravascular injection into the popliteal vessels. Appropriate technique and careful aspiration will decrease this risk.

Overdosage or *intravascular diffusion* can also cause symptoms of local anesthetic toxicity. Slow injection of local anesthetics decreases the incidence of this complication.

Pressure on the popliteal artery is rare and due to popliteal hematoma associated with arterial puncture and anticoagulant therapy.

Clinical Pearls

• Remember to block the saphenous nerve if the medial aspect of the lower limb is being operated on.

• Use a large volume of local anesthetic for the posterior approach; this results in better blockade due to the quantity of adipose tissue in the popliteal fossa.

• Stimulation of the biceps femoris muscle indicates too lateral a position of the needle with the posterior approach.

• A double-injection technique when using the lateral approach results in more consistent block rather than assuming the presence of a single nerve sheath, whereupon both nerves will be blocked if one is located.

Suggested reading

Hadzic A, Vloka JD. A comparison of the posterior versus lateral approaches to the block of the sciatic nerve in the popliteal fossa. Anesthesiology 1998; 88: 1480–1486.

Hadzic A, Vloka JD, Singson R, et al. A comparison of intertendinous and classical approaches to popliteal nerve block using magnetic resonance imaging simulation. Anesth Analg 2002; 94: 1321–1324.

Singelyn FJ, Aye F, Gouverneur JM. Continuous popliteal sciatic nerve block: an original technique to provide postoperative analgesia after foot surgery. Anesth Analg 1997; 84: 383–386.

Vloka JD, Hadzic A, April E, et al. The division of the sciatic nerve in the popliteal fossa: anatomical implications for popliteal nerve blockade. Anesth Analg 2001; 92: 215–217.

Zetlaoui PJ, Bouaziz H. Lateral approach to the sciatic nerve in the popliteal fossa. Anesth Analg 1998; 87: 79–82.

CHAPTER 26

Ankle block

Indications

Surgical—Surgical procedures on the forefoot, particularly the toes.
Therapeutic—Postamputation pain; diagnostic and therapeutic blocks for foot pain; postoperative pain relief.

Contraindications

Absolute
See Chapter 4.
Relative
Swollen ankle and leg tourniquet (necessitates higher blockade).

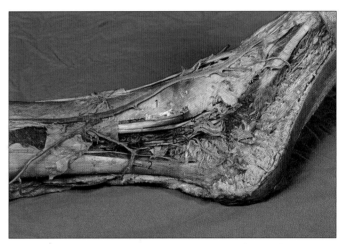

Figure 26.1 Cadaver structures of the medial aspect of the ankle illustrating anatomy pertinent to the ankle block. 1, Medial malleolus; 2, Achilles tendon; 3, tendon of tibialis posterior; 4, tendon of flexor digitorum longus; 5, posterior tibial artery and vein; 6, tibial nerve.

Anatomy

The ankle and foot are innervated by five nerves. One, the saphenous nerve, is the terminal branch of the femoral nerve, whereas the remaining four are branches of the sciatic nerve. These are the tibial nerve, the sural nerve, and the superficial and deep peroneal nerves.

The *tibial nerve* runs deep to the flexor retinaculum and posterior to the posterior tibial vein and artery, between the Achilles tendon and medial malleolus (Figs 26.1, 26.2). It divides into medial and lateral plantar nerves providing sensory innervation to the medial side of the sole of the foot and heel.

The tibial nerve provides motor supply to the intrinsic muscles of the foot. It is the largest nerve at the ankle, requiring the longest block onset, and thus should be blocked first.

The *deep peroneal nerve* runs deep to the extensor retinaculum and superficial to the tibia, lateral to the anterior tibial artery. It is bounded medially by the anterior tibial artery and tendon of the extensor hallucis longus muscle, and laterally by the extensors of the second toe. It provides sensory innervation to the tarsal and metatarsal joints and the first interdigital space.

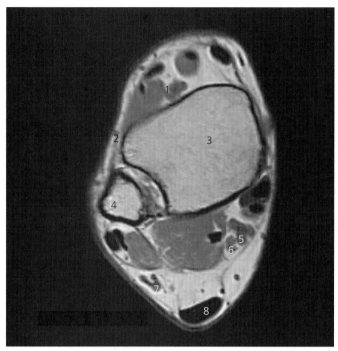

Figure 26.2 Axial T1-weighted MR image showing relevant anatomy of ankle. 1, Site of deep peroneal nerve; 2, superficial peroneal nerve; 3, tibia; 4, fibula; 5, posterior tibial artery; 6, tibial nerve; 7, sural nerve; 8, Achilles tendon.

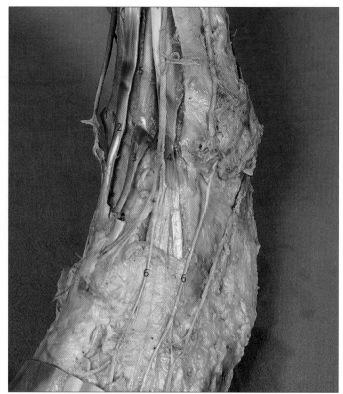

Figure 26.3 Cadaver structures of the ventral aspect of the ankle illustrating anatomy pertinent to the ankle block. 1, Medial malleolus; 2, tendon of tibialis anterior; 3, tendon of extensor hallucis longus; 4, tendon of extensor digitorum longus; 5, anterior tibial artery; 6, superficial peroneal nerve branches. The deep peroneal nerve is deep to fascia and cannot be seen here.

The *superficial peroneal nerve* travels distally with the peroneus brevis muscle, becoming superficial above the lateral malleolus, and runs over the dorsum of the foot, to which it provides sensory innervation (Figs 26.2, 26.3).

The *saphenous nerve* runs superficially with the great saphenous vein. It divides into terminal branches at the ankle. It provides sensory innervation to the medial aspect of the ankle and dorsum of the foot in a wedge shape toward the great toe.

The *sural nerve* runs superficially with the small saphenous vein and lies subcutaneously between the lateral malleolus and Achilles tendon (Figs 26.2, 26.4). It provides sensory innervation to the lateral aspect of the ankle and foot.

⬥ Surface anatomy

Important bony structures for the ankle block include the medial and lateral malleoli and the calcaneum. Other landmarks include the Achilles tendon, and on the ventral aspect of the ankle, the anterior tibial artery pulse and extensor hallucis longus tendons (Fig. 26.5). These tendons can be accentuated if the patient dorsiflexes the foot against resistance. A single needle insertion site at the midpoint of the intermalleolar line on the ventral aspect of the ankle is used for block of the superficial and deep peroneal nerves and saphenous nerve.

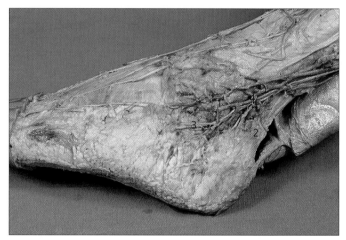

Figure 26.4 Cadaver structures of the lateral aspect of the ankle illustrating anatomy pertinent to the ankle block. 1, Lateral malleolus; 2, Achilles tendon; 3, sural nerve; 4, short saphenous vein.

Needle insertion for sural and tibial block is adjacent to the Achilles tendon, at the level of the superior aspect of the medial and lateral malleoli, respectively.

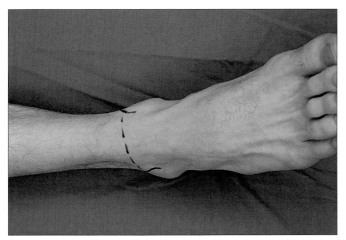

Figure 26.5 Landmarks for the ankle block include medial and lateral malleoli, intermalleolar line, dorsalis pedis pulse, and Achilles tendon.

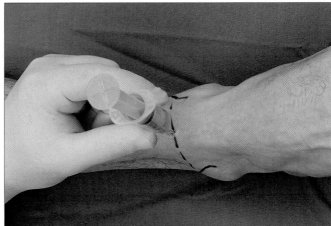

Figure 26.7 Deep peroneal nerve block technique. At the midpoint of the intermalleolar line and medial to the dorsalis pedis pulse, the needle is oriented perpendicular to the skin. On bony contact the needle is withdrawn slightly and injection is made.

✦ Technique

As for all regional anesthetic procedures, after checking that emergency equipment is complete and in working order, intravenous access, ECG, pulse oximetry, and blood pressure monitoring are established. Asepsis is observed.

Tibial nerve block

The block is performed by needle insertion on a line between medial malleolus and Achilles tendon (Fig. 26.6), just posterior to the tibial artery. If paresthesia is elicited, the needle should be withdrawn slightly and 5 mL of local anesthetic is injected. If paresthesia is not reported, the needle is advanced to the bone and withdrawn slightly, and 10 mL of local anesthetic injected.

Deep peroneal nerve block

To block the deep peroneal nerve, a needle is inserted between the extensor hallucis longus tendon and artery at the level of the intermalleolar line (Fig. 26.7). The needle is introduced perpendicular to the skin until bony contact is made, withdrawn slightly, and 4–5 mL of local anesthetic injected.

Saphenous nerve block

Saphenous nerve is blocked by subcutaneous injection passing medially from the insertion point of the deep peroneal nerve block toward the medial malleolus (Fig. 26.8), avoiding the saphenous vein. For this block, 4–5 mL of local anesthetic is adequate.

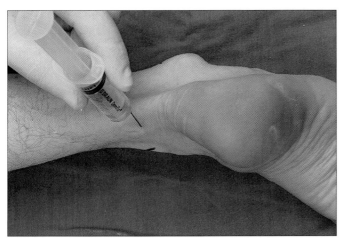

Figure 26.6 Tibial nerve block technique. The needle is inserted adjacent to the Achilles tendon and toward the superior aspect of the medial malleolus. On bony contact the needle is withdrawn and injection is made.

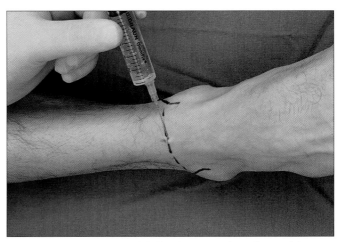

Figure 26.8 Saphenous nerve block technique. At the midpoint of the intermalleolar line a subcutaneous injection is made to the medial malleolus.

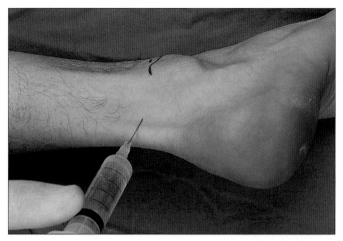

Figure 26.9 Superficial peroneal nerve block technique. At the midpoint of the intermalleolar line a subcutaneous injection is made to the lateral malleolus.

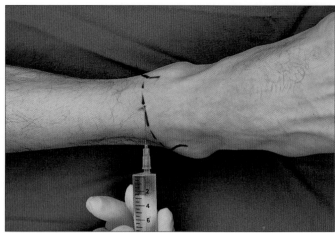

Figure 26.10 Sural nerve block technique. The needle is inserted adjacent to the Achilles tendon and toward the superior aspect of the lateral malleolus. On bony contact the needle is withdrawn and injection is made.

Superficial peroneal nerve block

The superficial peroneal nerve is blocked by a subcutaneous injection passing laterally from the insertion point of the deep peroneal nerve block toward the lateral malleolus (Fig. 26.9). For this block, 4–5 mL of local anesthetic is sufficient.

Sural nerve block

The sural nerve block is performed by needle insertion on a line between lateral malleolus and the Achilles tendon (Fig. 26.10). If paresthesia is reported, the needle is withdrawn slightly and injection made. Otherwise the needle is advanced until bony contact is made, withdrawn slightly, and the injection made.

The ankle block using the above technique uses three injection points. Alternatively, all five nerves can be blocked individually.

Clinical Pearls

• This block is relatively painful for the patient. It is worthwhile anesthetizing the skin with local anesthetic cream before injecting.

• For the tibial nerve block, it is best to place the foot to be injected over the opposite foot, with the medial malleolus uppermost. This gives good access to the nerve.

• This block is especially appropriate for the diabetic patient, who may also have multiple organ disease, requiring amputation of forefoot or toe(s).

• The tibial nerve can be located with a peripheral nerve stimulation technique; it is possible to place a catheter to provide continuous analgesia in its area of sensory innervation.

Suggested reading

Schurman DJ. Ankle-block anesthesia for foot surgery. Anesthesiology 1976; 4: 348–352.

CHAPTER 27
Paravertebral block

Indications

Surgical—Thoracic; breast; cholecystectomy; renal and ureteric; herniorrhaphy; appendicectomy; video-assisted thoracoscopic surgery; minimally invasive cardiac surgery.
Therapeutic—Acute pain management for fractured ribs and flail chest; intercostal neuralgia associated with osteoporotic vertebral fractures; liver capsular pain after blunt abdominal trauma; acute and chronic postherpetic neuralgia; postamputation pain; chronic benign and tumor-related pain; prolonged postoperative analgesia (continuous technique).

Contraindications

Absolute
See Chapter 4.
Relative
Hemorrhagic diathesis; anticoagulation treatment; distorted anatomy (e.g. kyphoscoliosis or previous thoracic surgery).

Anatomy

The paravertebral space is a wedge-shaped area on both sides of the vertebral column (Fig. 27.1). The boundaries of the space are posteriorly, the superior costotransverse ligament;

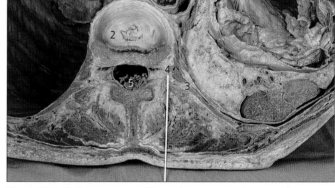

Figure 27.1 Cadaver structures illustrating anatomy relevant to the paravertebral block. 1, Spinous process; 2, vertebral body; 3, transverse process; 4, paravertebral space; 5, spinal canal.

laterally, the posterior intercostal membrane; and anteriorly, the parietal pleura. At the base of the triangle (medially) is the posterolateral aspect of the vertebra, disc, and intervertebral foramen (Fig. 27.2). Contents of the paravertebral space include fatty tissue, intercostal vessels, spinal (intercostal) nerve, dorsal ramus, rami communicantes, and sympathetic chain (anteriorly). The paravertebral space is continuous medially with the epidural space and laterally with the intercostal space. The inferior limit of this space occurs at the origins of the psoas major muscle. The superior limit extends into the cervical region.

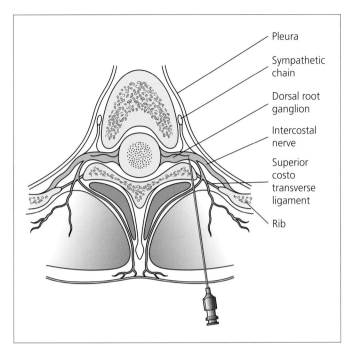

Figure 27.2 Anatomy of the paravertebral space.

⬥ Surface anatomy

The main landmarks for the paravertebral block are the spinous and transverse processes. Identification of the appropriate vertebral level for blockade is facilitated by knowledge of dermatomes and anatomic landmarks that suggest vertebral level (Fig. 27.3). The spinous process of C7 (vertebrae prominens) is prominent and does not move with neck flexion. The spine and inferior angle of the scapula lie at the T3 and T7 vertebral levels, respectively.

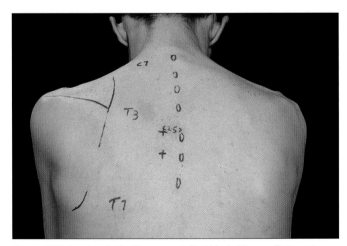

Figure 27.3 Landmarks for the paravertebral block. The needle insertion point is 2.5 cm lateral to the spinous process. Approximate vertebral levels can be obtained by positioning of the spine and inferior angle of the scapula and the vertebrae prominens (C7).

Technique

As for all regional anesthetic procedures, after checking that emergency equipment is complete and in working order, intravenous access, ECG, pulse oximetry, and blood pressure monitoring are established. Asepsis is observed.

The patient is placed in the sitting or lateral position with the head in the flexed position and the back arched. Choose which dermatomes will be involved in the operative field. The spinous processes are palpated and marked with a skin marker. A point 2.5 cm lateral to the spinous processes is marked.

The needle insertion point is infiltrated with local anesthetic using a 25-G needle. An 18-G Tuohy needle is inserted perpendicular to the skin until contact is made with the transverse process (Fig. 27.4). This usually occurs 2–4 cm from the skin.

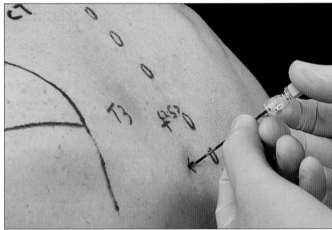

Figure 27.4 Paravertebral block technique. The epidural needle is inserted perpendicular to the skin until contact with the transverse process.

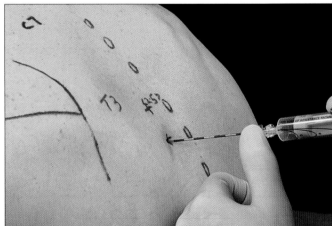

Figure 27.5 Paravertebral block technique. The needle is 'walked' over the transverse process and advanced until a loss of resistance is identified.

The location of the transverse process is critical in the performance of this block. If this contact is not made, it is likely that the needle lies between the transverse processes. The needle should be withdrawn and redirected in a caudal or cephalic direction (Fig. 27.5). Once the transverse process is identified, the needle is withdrawn and redirected in a cephalic direction to 'walk' over the transverse process.

The paravertebral space is usually found 1–1.5 cm deep to the transverse process. It is imperative that the needle should not be advanced beyond this point because there is a risk of pleural puncture. A subtle 'click' or loss of resistance is

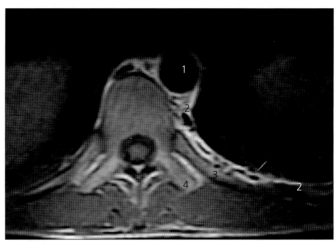

Figure 27.7 Axial T1-weighted MR image showing spread of contrast laterally below the ninth rib. 1, aorta; 2, intracostal contrast spread; 3, ninth rib; 4, T9 transverse process.

usually felt as the needle passes through the costotransverse ligament.

Incremental injections of local anesthetic (5 mL) are made with repeated aspiration. For a single-injection multisegment block, the volume used should be 15–25 mL. While the onset of analgesia is within minutes after injection of local anesthetic, up to 20 min is typically required for surgical anesthesia. If a catheter is required this is passed after the bolus injection. The required length is 3–4 cm in the paravertebral space.

Local anesthetic solution injected into the paravertebral space may remain localized, spread to the ipsilateral paravertebral spaces above and below the injection site (Fig. 27.6), pass laterally through the intercostal space (Fig. 27.7), or spread medially through the epidural space or across the vertebral bodies. Thermographic studies have demonstrated that 15 mL of bupivacaine 0.5% produces a somatic block of five dermatomes and a sympathetic block over eight dermatomes. Little is known regarding the factors that influence spread.

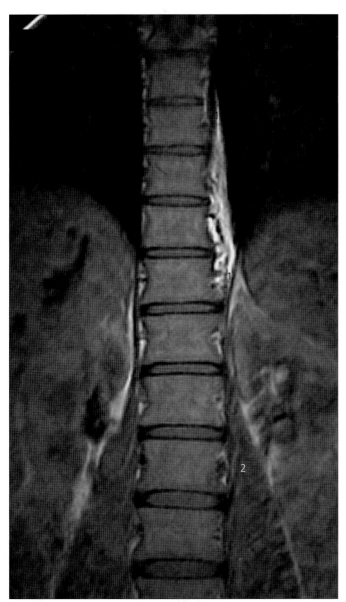

Figure 27.6 Coronal T1-weighted MR image showing cephalad and caudad spread of 20 mL of contrast injected below transverse process of T10. 1, Contrast spread; 2 psoas muscle.

◈ Adverse effects

Hematoma.

Hypotension due to sympathetic block is decreased compared with centroneuroaxial techniques.

Local anesthetic toxicity is rare; avoid by frequent aspiration.

Epidural or subarachnoid injection: bilateral anesthesia suggests an epidural or intrathecal injection; avoid by preventing any medial orientation of the needle. Bilateral anesthesia may also occur by spread of local anesthetic across the vertebral bodies.

Pneumothorax is unlikely with correct technique (0.5% incidence).

Clinical Pearls

• Simple and easy to learn with a low incidence of complications.

• Compared with thoracic epidural techniques, it maintains hemodynamic stability, bladder sensation, and lower limb motor power. Promotes early mobilization.

• Reliably blocks the posterior primary ramus, unlike the intercostal technique.

Suggested reading

Karmakar MK. Thoracic paravertebral block. Anesthesiology 2001; 95: 771–780.

Naja Z, Lönnqvist PA. Somatic paravertebral blockade. Incidence of failed block and complications. Anaesthesia 2001; 56: 1184–1188.

Richardson J, Lönnqvist PA. Thoracic paravertebral block. Br J Anaesth 1998; 81: 230–238.

CHAPTER 28

Intercostal block

⬥ Indications

Surgical—Upper abdominal and thoracic superficial procedures; insertion of thoracotomy and gastrostomy tubes.
Therapeutic—Postoperative pain therapy after upper abdominal and thoracic procedures; intercostal neuralgia; painful conditions after rib fractures or contusions of chest wall; pleuritic pain; postherpetic neuralgia; tumor-related pain.

⬥ Contraindications

Absolute
See Chapter 4.
Relative
Hemorrhagic diathesis; anticoagulation treatment; and chronic obstructive lung disease.

⬥ Anatomy

The intercostal nerves comprise the ventral rami of T1 to T11. The 12th thoracic nerve is called the subcostal nerve. The intercostal nerves contribute and receive sympathetic fibers. Shortly after exit from the intervertebral foramina, the dorsal rami become a posterior cutaneous branch to skin and muscles in the paravertebral region (Fig. 28.1). At the angle of the ribs, a lateral cutaneous and a collateral branch arise. The collateral

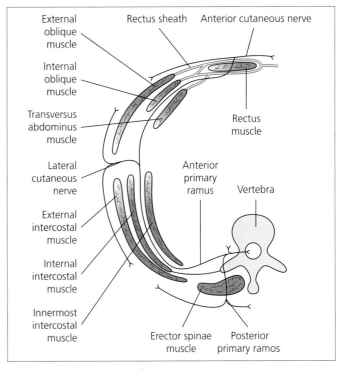

Figure 28.1 Typical intercostal nerve.

branch follows the lower border of the space in the same intermuscular interval as the main trunk, which it may or may not rejoin before it is distributed as an additional anterior cutaneous branch. The lateral branch accompanies the main trunk for a time before piercing the intercostal muscles

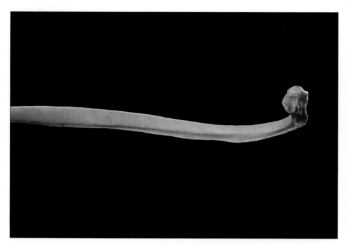

Figure 28.2 The interior lower edge of the ribs provides a channel for the intercostal nerve and its companion artery and vein. The nerve lies just behind the lower border of the rib. Near the midaxillary line the groove becomes less well defined, and the nerve migrates away from the rib.

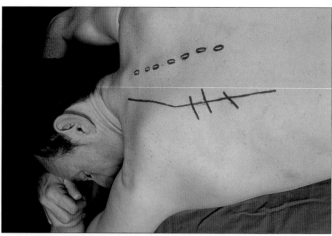

Figure 28.3 Landmarks for the intercostal block. The patient lies in the prone position with the arms abducted above the head. The spinal musculature is identified and marked laterally. The inferior border of the ribs are marked where they cross this muscle mass.

obliquely. The main trunk continues anteriorly as the anterior cutaneous branch.

The interior lower edge of the ribs provides a channel for the intercostal nerve and its companion artery and vein. The nerve lies just behind the lower border of the rib. Near the midaxillary line the groove becomes less well defined, and the nerve migrates away from the rib (Fig. 28.2). The structures between skin and intercostal nerve vary depending on body wall location on the nerve's path. At the back of the chest the nerve lies between the pleura and the posterior intercostal membrane (extension of internal intercostal muscle), but in most of its course it runs between the internal intercostal muscles and the intercostalis intimi. Where the latter muscles are absent, the nerve lies in contact with the parietal pleura. In the intercostal groove the vein lies superior, with the artery and nerve more inferiorly. This relation is not consistent, particularly in the paravertebral region.

Surface anatomy

Important bony structures relevant to the intercostal nerve block include the thoracic spinous processes, paraspinal muscles, posterior angulation of ribs, spine, and inferior tip of scapula. The lateral edge of the paraspinal muscles are identified and marked. This is at the posterior angle of the ribs. These lines angle medially in the upper thoracic region so as to parallel the medial edge of the scapula. The midline spinous processes are also marked. The inferior edge of ribs are palpated and marked. At the intersection of lines are the needle insertion points (Fig. 28.3).

Technique

As for all regional anesthetic procedures, after checking that emergency equipment is complete and in working order, intravenous access, ECG, pulse oximetry, and blood pressure monitoring are established. Asepsis is observed.

In the posterior approach the patient lies in a prone or lateral position. The prone position is particularly favored if bilateral blocks are to be performed. The operator stands behind the patient. A pillow is placed under the abdomen to reduce the lumbar lordosis and to accentuate the intercostal spaces posteriorly. The arms should be allowed to hang down from the edge of the block table to permit the scapula to rotate as far laterally as possible.

The needle insertion point is infiltrated with local anesthetic using a 25-G needle. The index and third finger of left hand retract skin up and over rib. A 15-mm 25-G needle is introduced in 20° cephalad orientation through the skin between the tip of the retracting fingers, and advanced until it contacts rib (Fig. 28.4). The left hand now holds needle hub and shaft between the thumb, index finger, and middle finger. The left-hand hypothenar eminence is firmly placed against the patient's back. The needle and syringe move as a whole. This allows maximal control of needle depth as the left hand 'walks' the needle off the inferior margin of the rib and into the intercostal groove. At a distance of 2–4 mm past the edge of the rib, 3–5 mL of local anesthetic is injected after aspiration (Fig. 28.5). The intercostal block may also be performed in the midaxillary line, but there is risk of not blocking the lateral cutaneous branch.

Continuous intercostal techniques have been described.

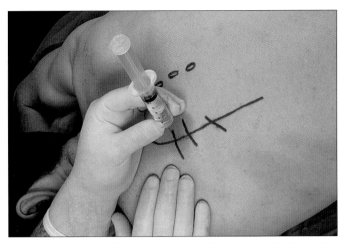

Figure 28.4 Intercostal block technique: introducing the needle. The index and third finger retract skin up and over rib. The needle is introduced in 20° cephalad orientation and advanced until it contacts rib.

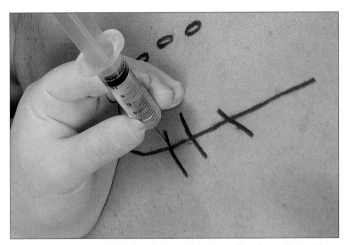

Figure 28.5 Intercostal block technique: injection of local anesthetic. The left hand now holds needle hub and shaft between the thumb, index finger, and middle finger. The left-hand hypothenar eminence is firmly placed against the patient's back. The needle and syringe move as a whole. This allows maximal control of needle depth as the left hand 'walks' the needle off the inferior margin of the rib and into the intercostal groove. At a distance of 2–4 mm past the edge of the rib, 3–5 mL of local anesthetic is injected.

◈ Adverse effects

Bruising.

Neural injuries are extremely rare.

Local anesthetic toxicity due to intravascular injection into the intercostal vessels is decreased by careful aspiration. Overdosage or intravascular diffusion can cause symptoms of local anesthetic toxicity. Slow injection will decrease the incidence of this complication.

Pneumothorax, which occurs in less than 1% of blocks, can be minimized by appropriate technique.

Clinical Pearls

• Individuals should develop a consistent technique of hand and needle control for this block.

• Patient positioning improves success in obese patients.

• If multiple levels are to be blocked then sedation is mandatory.

Suggested reading

Shanti CM, Carlin AM, Tyburski JG. Incidence of pneumothorax from intercostal nerve block for analgesia in rib fractures. J Trauma 2001; 51: 536–539.

CHAPTER 29

Inguinal field block

Local anesthesia is used frequently for inguinal hernia repair. This surgery is more commonly being performed as an ambulatory procedure, and regional anesthesia may offer advantages for this; it may also be the technique of choice in patients with intercurrent diseases. The technique involves the blocking of the ilioinguinal, iliohypogastric, and genitofemoral nerves in combination with subcutaneous injection.

This chapter describes techniques for blocking these nerves, which can also be used individually for postoperative pain relief and diagnostic or therapeutic blocks for groin pain, as well as for superficial surgery.

ANATOMY

The anterolateral abdominal wall comprises three musculo-aponeurotic layers. From deep to superficial these are the tranversus abdominis, internal oblique, and external oblique. A neurovascular plane exists between the first and second of these layers. The subcostal (T12), iliohypogastric (L1), and ilioinguinal (L1) nerves emerge from the upper part of the lateral border of the psoas major muscle. They pass laterally in front of quadratus lumborum to enter the neurovascular plane, where they slope down and around the abdominal wall.

The *subcostal nerve* ends by innervating the lower part of rectus abdominis muscle and the skin overlying it. Its lateral cutaneous branch innervates the skin of the anterior buttock between the iliac crest and greater trochanter.

The *iliohypogastric nerve* gives a branch that innervates an area of buttock behind that innervated by the subcostal. The iliohypogastric nerve pierces the internal oblique muscle above the anterior superior iliac spine, slopes downward between internal oblique and external oblique muscles (Fig. 29.1), then pierces the external oblique aponeurosis 3 cm above the superficial inguinal ring, and ends by innervating skin over the lower part of rectus abdominis and front of pubis.

The *ilioinguinal nerve* represents the collateral branch of the iliohypogastric nerve, with which it runs parallel. It pierces the transversus abdominis muscle close to the anterior superior anterior iliac spine to lie between the transversus abdominis and internal oblique muscles (Fig. 29.2). It subsequently enters the inguinal canal, travels inferomedially, and emerges from the superficial inguinal ring.

SURFACE ANATOMY

Important bony structures for the inguinal block include the anterior superior iliac spine and pubic tubercle. The needle insertion site for ilioinguinal and iliohypogastric nerve blocks is 1 cm medial and 1 cm inferior to the anterior superior iliac spine. The pubic tubercle can be palpated 3 cm from the midline. The needle insertion site for block of the genital branch of genitofemoral nerve is 2 cm laterally and 2 cm cephalad from the pubic tubercle.

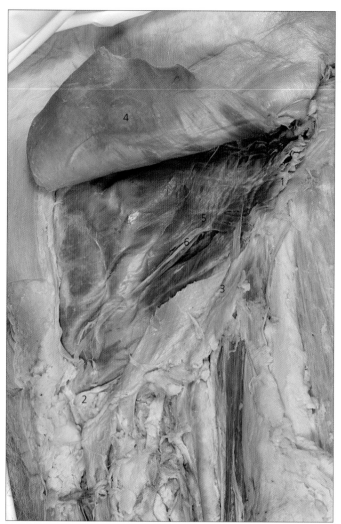

Figure 29.1 Cadaver structures illustrating anatomy pertinent to the inguinal block technique. 1, Anterior superior iliac spine; 2, pubic tubercle; 3, inguinal ligament; 4, external oblique aponeurosis (retracted); 5, internal oblique muscle; 6, iliohypogastric nerve.

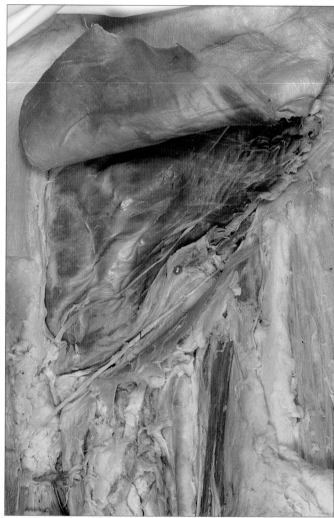

Figure 29.2 The external oblique close to the inguinal ligament is now retracted, illustrating the ilioinguinal nerve. 1, Ilioinguinal nerve.

ILIOINGUINAL NERVE BLOCK

⬥ Indications

Surgical—As part of field block for groin surgery.
Therapeutic—Postoperative pain relief; diagnostic block for groin pain; neuralgia, especially after hernia repair.

⬥ Contraindications

Absolute
See Chapter 4.

Relative
Large hernias, especially scrotal; bleeding diathesis; and morbid obesity.

⬥ Anatomy

See p. 141.

⬥ Technique

As for all regional anesthetic procedures, after checking that emergency equipment is complete and in working order,

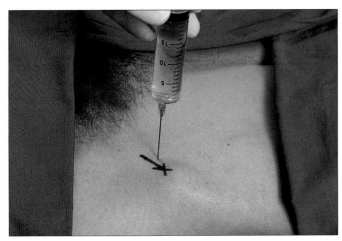

Figure 29.3 Inguinal block technique: ilioinguinal and iliohypogastric nerves. The needle insertion point is 1 cm medial and 1 cm inferior from the anterior superior iliac spine (above the inguinal ligament). The needle is inserted perpendicular to the skin.

intravenous access, ECG, pulse oximetry, and blood pressure monitoring are established. Asepsis is observed.

The patient lies supine. The operator stands at the side to be anesthetized. The ilioinguinal and iliohypogastric nerve are anesthetized at a single injection site (Fig. 29.3). A 35-mm 21-G needle is inserted through the skin 1 cm medial and 1 cm inferior to the anterior superior iliac spine. The needle is held lightly between the fingers and slowly advanced in an incremental fashion; the 'clicks' of the abdominal wall are best appreciated with this technique. Resting the ulnar border of the injecting hand on the patient can help steady it, to prevent overshooting the target.

On piercing the external oblique muscle, 6–8 mL of local anesthetic are injected to anesthetize the iliohypogastric nerve. Advancing the needle further pierces the internal oblique muscle. Local anesthetic (increments of 2–5 mL within the calculated maximum allowable) is injected here to anesthetize the ilioinguinal nerve.

Injection is also made subcutaneously toward the ilium until bony contact is made to anesthetize the lateral cutaneous branch of the subcostal nerve. A transverse subcutaneous injection toward the midline is also made to block further branches from the subcostal nerve.

GENITOFEMORAL NERVE BLOCK

Indications

Surgical—As part of field block for groin surgery.
Therapeutic—Postoperative pain relief; diagnostic block for groin pain; neuralgia, especially after hernia repair.

Contraindications

Absolute
See Chapter 4.
Relative
Large hernias, especially scrotal; bleeding diathesis; anticoagulation therapy; and morbid obesity.

Anatomy

The genitofemoral nerve has its origin from the second lumbar nerve, with a contribution from the lower branch of the first lumbar nerve. It emerges on to the anterior surface of psoas major muscle, cephalad to the inguinal ligament. The femoral branch follows the femoral artery to pass deep to the inguinal ligament. The genital branch enters the spermatic cord (round ligament), innervates the cremaster muscle and anterolateral scrotum, and passes through the superficial inguinal canal close to the pubic tubercle.

Technique

The genital branch is blocked by inserting a 35-mm 23-G needle 2 cm lateral and 2 cm superior to the pubic tubercle (Fig. 29.4). The needle is passed medially until the pubic tubercle is contacted, withdrawn slightly, and injection of 4–5 mL of local anesthetic made in a fan-shaped manner. A vertical injection in the midline at the pubis is made to block overlapping innervation from the contralateral side.

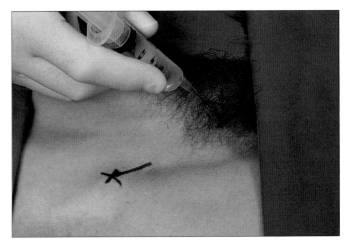

Figure 29.4 Inguinal block technique: genitofemoral nerve. The needle insertion point is 2 cm lateral and 2 cm superior from the pubic tubercle. The needle is inserted toward the pubic tubercle. On bony contact the needle is withdrawn and injection is made.

Inguinal hernia repair requires, in addition to these nerve blocks, a subcutaneous injection of local anesthetic at the incision site (5–6 mL) and intraoperative block of the neck of the hernial sac (3–4 mL), because intestine has a separate sensory (sympathetic) nerve supply.

Inguinal hernia repair can also be performed using an infiltration technique (normally done by the surgeon).

◈ Adverse effects

Hematoma.

Block of the lateral cutaneous nerve of thigh (close to needle insertion site).

Local anesthetic toxicity: take care with total dose of drug because large volumes of local anesthetic may be needed, especially in obese patients.

Clinical Pearls

- Gives excellent conditions for hernia repair.
- Associated with high incidence of patient satisfaction.
- Ideal for 'day case' procedures.
- Less useful for very large and recurrent hernias.
- Needs cooperative colleagues.
- Nerve stimulation not necessary.
- Calculate total safe dose of local anesthetic and do not exceed it.

Suggested reading

Amid PK, Shulman AG, Lichtenstein IL. Local anaesthesia for inguinal hernia repair: step-by-step procedure. Ann Surg 1994; 220: 735–737.

Index